# Praise for *Crack the Code*

"Transformational … As a professional athlete, broadcaster, and father, I've experienced the power of motivation from a number of viewpoints. **Crack The Code** does a fantastic job of demonstrating the force of social and emotional motivators in creating a healthy lifestyle in men over 50. The stories humanize its strategies and show that positive behavior, and its benefits, is within every man's reach. An incredibly important read for 50+ men and the people that love them."

> — **Bill Clement, Two-Time Stanley Cup Champi**
> **broadcaster, speaker and author of *Every Day***
> ***Crossing Gorges on T***

"**Crack The Code** nails it. Lou Bezich p compelling reason to re-think our lifestyle health offers a winning strategy to get th out of life. It's an incredibly important wake-up call delivered in an uncomplicated and stimulating fashion, which will relate to men. It helped me realize that sustaining healthy behavior is a team sport and that's why I plan to share this book with the most important people in my life, my family. You should too."

> — **Ron Jaworski, Pro-Bowl Quarterback,**
> **CEO, Ron Jaworski Golf Management, broadcaster,**
> **and author of *The Games That Changed the Game***

"**Crack The Code** is an essential read not for just men over 50, but also for people who care for and want to understand men over 50. It is a blend of tactical, strategic, and practical hints and cultural concepts.

Reading it is an investment of time that will yield a lifetime of dividends."

— **Jim Florio, Former Governor of New Jersey,**
**Partner, Florio, Perrucci, Steinhardt & Fader**

"Lou's insights are invaluable—and they come at a crucial time in the history of the health care system of the United States. Families, businesses, governments, and taxpayers all confront exploding health care costs. The principal source of these exploding costs relates to treatment of chronic disease, and no strategy for reducing these costs will succeed if it is not grounded in a clear understanding of behavioral characteristics—what makes people tick. This book deftly blends academic research, Lou's strategic experience, and clearly written common sense ideas. I hope Lou further enriches our understanding by expanding his scope to other groups in our culture and community."

— **Rob Andrews, CEO Health Transformation Alliance**
**and Former US Congressman**

"A call to action … Lou Bezich reminds all of us over 50 what we have to live for and where to find the fulfillment to sustain a healthy lifestyle. *Crack The Code* is a dynamite combination of research, stories, and practical advice that shows that the inspiration that drives happiness and health is right in front of us. It is a code that my wife, Janet, and I subscribe to, as we believe in tiger synergy of mind, body, and fitness. If you want to feel Invincible this is a book that you'll want to read and share with the most important people in your life."

— **Vince Papale, Motivational Speaker, NFL alum,**
**subject of the Disney movie *Invincible*, and author**
**of *Be Invincible! A Playbook for Reaching Your Full Potential***
**by Vince Papale and Janet Cantwell-Papale with Time Vandehey.**
**He also authored *The Last Laugh - Vision to Victory*, with his**
**teammate and lifelong friend, Dennis Franks**

"A winning strategy … Lou Bezich has taken on the impossible task of motivating men over 50 to live healthy and created a highly successful model that will appeal to even the most cynical and stubborn among us. He's leveraged the power of emotion and provided easy-to-use strategies that every man can grasp. In my playing career, I saw how motivated players could achieve success when others didn't give them a chance. Lou's book will do the same for you. Read it!"

— **Bernie Parent, Member, Hockey Hall of Fame, Two-Time Stanley Cup Champion, Vezina Trophy and Conn Smythe Trophy winner. Named one of the "100 Greatest NHL Players" in history (2017)**

"If you are a man over 50, *Crack The Code* should be required reading. Louis Bezich examines the so-called "golden years" in ways that are both helpful and hopeful."

— **Ray Didinger, 94 WIP Sports Radio**

"Lou Bezich has indeed cracked the secret code among all too macho men! Every guy knows that going to the doctor makes you a sissy and that sharing intimate health details is akin to fumbling the football on the one-yard line. Bezich "tackles" these tightly held myths and turns the game around. He knows that you cannot improve the health of a population—in this case reluctant men—without their engagement in the process. He has written the playbook that all men need to read and to embrace. Maybe men will even share the playbook with their spouse, girlfriend, and grown daughters. Imagine the improvement in outcomes we could achieve!! Kudos to Bezich for grabbing this fumble and running it all the way down the field for a true touchdown for health! I hope every guy will read this great book."

— **David B. Nash MD, MBA, Founding Dean, Jefferson College of Population Health, Phila, PA**

"In *Crack The Code*, Lou has integrated several perspectives from motivation science intending to enhance the wellbeing of men over fifty. All people can benefit from this approach, but we (men over fifty) are great at ignoring our health needs. Men stand to gain substantially longer lives, and higher quality of life years for the years we live if we learn to attend to our motivational needs while making health related changes."

— **Dr. Geoffrey Williams, Professor of Medicine, Psychiatry, and Psychology at the University of Rochester Medical Center**

"This book tackles a tough topic ... how to get men engaged in their own health. It's accessible, fun to read, and extremely well researched. The book is based on both real-life experience from the author, a national survey, and input from experts around the country. Men who want to get healthier and anyone concerned about the health of a man in their life should buy and read this book."

— **Jeff Brenner MD, Senior Vice President-Clinical Redesign, United Healthcare Community & State, Mac Arthur Genius Award Recipient, Founder-Camden Coalition of Healthcare Providers**

"As a 63 year-old man, working in a high-stress, long-hours job, I have experienced firsthand the benefits that living a healthy lifestyle can provide. Personally, I view a structured exercise program as a powerful antidote to the stress and adversity inherent in my life. *Crack the Code* not only provides both the evidence that can help motivate older men (everyone really) to begin taking the steps necessary to improve their quality of life, it also offers a concrete, manageable roadmap to make this journey a reality. Should be mandatory reading for anyone looking to extend their life expectancy and improve their quality of existence."

— **Don Borden, President, Camden County College**

# CRACK
## THE CODE

## 10 Proven Secrets
that Motivate Healthy Behavior
and Inspire Fulfillment
in Men Over 50

## LOUIS BEZICH

SOMO Press

CRACK THE CODE: *10 Proven Secrets that Motivate Healthy Behavior
and Inspire Fulfillment in Men Over 50*
by Louis Bezich

Published by

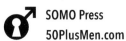 **SOMO Press**
50PlusMen.com

PO Box 151, Collingswood, NJ 08108

ISBN: 978-1-7325528-0-7 (print)
ISBN: 978-1-7325528-1-4 (ebook)
Library of Congress Control Number: 2018908121

Editing: Cynde Christie, cynde_christie@yahoo.com
Book Design: Nick Zelinger, www.NZGraphics.com

10 9 8 7 6 5 4 3 2 1

HEALTH & FITNESS  1. General   2. Men's Health   3. Healthy Living

First Edition

Printed in the United States

Disclaimer: This book is not intended to be a substitute for the medical advice
of a licensed physician. The reader should always consult with their doctor in
any matters relating to his/her health.

*I dedicate this book to my father, Anthony M. Bezich, who passed away on December 10, 2017, during the final stages of this book. His influence is present throughout this work, and he has been an inspiration to my family and me. He truly exemplified the power of social motivation.*

# Contents

———————————————— **II** ————————————————

# Table of Figures

# Introduction

Too many men 50, and older, live in a perpetual state of irony. They want what's best for themselves and their families, but their actions suggest otherwise. When shopping for a new car or a vacation, they'll search endlessly for the best value. Time and effort goes into all sorts of priorities, from their grandchildren to their favorite sports team. The last thing they want is to be a burden. They grew up seeing themselves as the providers and guardians of others.

Yet, when it comes to the one common denominator with the greatest potential to affect the fulfillment of this aspiration, attending to their health, men ignore the opportunity. Their behavior is inconsistent, as they are seemingly unaware that health is a prerequisite for these goals. The results speak volumes.

In general, men are less healthy than women are and have a shorter life expectancy (75 years vs. 80 years for women) (Xu & Borders, 2003). Twice as many men as women die each year from heart attacks, and the rates of other major diseases such as stroke, diabetes, and chronic lung disease are all higher in men (US Department of Health and Human Services). Finally, men visit their doctor for preventative care half as often as women do, and all these differences become more acute as men pass the 50-year mark (Galdas, Cheater & Marshall, 2005).

I will leave the historical causes of this situation to others. My focus is on the future and, more specifically, the search for a new approach to men's health, one with sustainability and the power to ignite cultural reform. My interest centers on the significant impact of behavior on health and, more specifically, the sources of motivation and social factors necessary to sustain a healthy lifestyle.

Using a combination of survey research and personal interviews, I document the sources of motivation and the common traits among healthily behaving 50+ men and translate the results into concrete strategies and actions that form a 10-step motivational blueprint. Real-life stories from my men illustrate the findings and provide deeper meaning and purpose. In addition, I share my own personal experiences to add further dimension and inspiration for my brothers who continue to struggle with the climb up the mountain of healthy living.

My hope is that by researching and writing about a sub-set of 50+ men who buck the trend by leading a healthy life, I will produce insights and strategies that are usable by this population and others. I suspect that the women and partners who love these men will have an interest in what I've learned, as well as the physicians and clinicians who treat them, the companies that insure their health, and the policy-makers who control the systems that regulate their care.

As a healthcare executive, husband, father, grandfather, part-time professor, and author with a passion for health and fitness, my devotion developed through a lifetime of experiences that included the death of an unborn child, divorce, single parenthood, and professional challenges. Diet and exercise became my antidote to surviving the tough times and ultimately flourishing. Decades later, what started as a coping mechanism for an ambitious 20-something kid has grown into a devotion that drives this 60-something man to share my experience, promote socially-based motivation models, and advocate for a new culture of men's health.

While I reference the abundance of academic research on behavior change, primarily from the field of psychology, to support my model, my goal is adoption. With over 40 years in management, my interests are practical, not academic. They reside in the need for leadership on a topic which is both personal to me and yet extremely public. We live in a country with the greatest health care available on earth, but our own behavior results in an alarming state of poor health, most evident in men over 50.

The existing approaches to men's health have failed. If anything, our experience is trending in the wrong direction. *Crack the Code* offers a different approach—one that reaches far upstream from the medicine, diets, and exercise fads that dominate our culture for a model grounded in the most powerful of all motivations. For it is only through a meaningful alignment of motivation and behavior that we discover a model to provide the scalability and sustainability needed by the cohort of 50+ men and others.

I believe that we are at a crossroads. I see hope for this new model of men's health in a joining together of factors, ranging from economic factors that have extended employment opportunities for older men and technology that make socializing easier for men, to a mounting recognition of the impact of social determinants on health. Together, I believe that these factors, along with the tenacity of the aging baby boomer, can spur a counter-culture, much like that produced by this generation decades ago.

Giving further hope is the methodology I've used to create a new, socially based model for men's health. Three overarching strategies form the platform found in the chapters that follow:

## 1. The Messenger

Leading theories of psychology indicate that the recipient of a message is more receptive and more likely to adopt the behavior promoted in the message if the messenger is like them. I designed my survey data and personal interviews from 50+ men to add a level of credibility and relatedness for readers, and greatly increase the potential for men to adopt healthy behaviors.

## 2. The Moment

The timing of the message is also critical to receptivity and adoption. Healthy men suggest that there are moments when men observe and most directly feel the repercussions of unhealthy behavior, whether the death of a loved one, losing one's breath after climbing stairs, or simply finding that their pants don't fit. During these moments, the message of healthy behavior is more apt to strike a chord. Incorporating such decisive moments in this work offers a strategic tool to further increase adoption.

### 3. The Message Framing

How we frame the message is the third critical attribute. A man's core values and the advancement of his life's priorities are emotions that play to his strongest intrinsic motivations. This powerful framing is essential to the task of triggering behavior change and another tactic that differentiates my model.

Yes, 50+ men can enjoy a healthy lifestyle and the benefits that it provides. Come, brothers, let me show you the way. You deserve it!

# 1

# The Case for Motivation

"IT SOUNDS LIKE YOU'RE asking me why I want to be healthy," he said, brow furrowing. "I don't quite—understand." Steve had arrived at a southern New Jersey research facility about an hour before. He passed a variety of screening inquiries confirming that he leads a healthy lifestyle and agreed to answer questions about his health behaviors. Eight other 50+men of broad life experiences joined him.

As an initial step in my research, I assembled two identical groups of men, one in New Jersey and one in San Francisco. Both groups exhibited positive health behaviors as defined by Dr. David Nash, dean of the School of Population Health of the Thomas Jefferson University, as a reasonable BMI (body mass index), regular exercise, consumption of fresh fruits and vegetables, abstinence from smoking, and the use of a seat belt. Their age and these criteria were the basis for their selection.

While many health services occur in the confines of hospitals and medical offices, health care providers have long understood that successful health outcomes mold more significantly in the home, gym, and grocery store. Steve and the other study participants shared what inspired them to live their healthy lifestyles. On the surface, Steve and his colleagues seemed to connect what they value most in life: their spouses, children, grandchildren, vocations, and hobbies, to the importance of healthy practices. Several explained how they integrated these valued relationships into their diet and exercise routines to create a mutually supportive lifestyle that helps sustain their health.

Besides screening questions for a nationwide survey of men like themselves, I wanted to uncover their secret sauce. I wanted to know how they think about their life and what's behind their healthy lifestyle. Why is it that they can accomplish what so many men their age can't? Moreover, once gaining these insights, how could I create a model for other 50+ men (or all men, for that matter) to follow? While 50+ men in general are the least healthy group in the nation, these men proved that a healthy lifestyle at 50+ was possible (CDC, 2003).

My question was, "How do they do it?" and, even more precisely, "Where do they get their motivation?" My search for these answers included the nationwide survey that I was screening with Steve and his colleagues, as well as personal interviews.

## A Wake-up Call for 50+ Men

Remarkable, isn't it? By far, we spend more money on health care than any other country in the world, and yet the general health of Americans ranks well below most leading industrialized nations (CDC, 2003). To think that despite all this investment in science, technology, pharmacology, and medical education that what's most important, what makes the biggest difference, is our ability to live healthily. Yet, as a society, we struggle with high rates of obesity and chronic illnesses, both highly influenced by lifestyle (TFAH, RWJF, 2017).

This is not to say that Americans are unaware of the problem. God knows the bookstores contain many diet and exercise books, gyms of all types dot the country, and an endless stream of infomercials promote exercise equipment, while health care providers promote disease prevention and offer instruction on healthy behavior.

## Health Behaviors Need Not Be Costly

I am lucky to have a career that has enabled me to provide for my family and given me access to modest resources, such as a gym membership. For that, I am grateful. However, it is important to note that neither the social or the behavioral dimensions of a healthy lifestyle necessarily represent a costly proposition. A little creativity can go a long way.

Socially, I've often taken a nice walk in the park, enjoyed a glass of inexpensive wine, and enjoyed conversation, as ways to make the social connections I sought with my significant others. Over the years, I've also availed myself of public concerts, festivals, and/or a stroll through the city as a vehicle for socializing. Family gatherings are certainly a traditional means to reinforce your priorities, without breaking the bank.

As for behavior, long before I became a gym rat, I was running the streets and sidewalks, doing push-ups in my basement, and taking advantage of public recreational resources to meet my exercise needs. As for diet, there is significant economy in healthy foods, when compared to the demons of fast food. While access to healthy food can sometimes be an obstacle, particularly in some urban areas, more and more farmers' markets are popping-up, providing reasonable access to fruits, vegetables, and healthy food products.

Granted, nothing is easy in life and this includes your health behaviors. My point is to acknowledge that men bring varied levels of resources to bear on their goal of lifestyle change. Whatever your situation, my experience is that there are opportunities to meet your needs. It requires some innovative thinking, but is certainly within the reach of every man who aspires to live healthily. Health insurers now have all sorts of incentives for healthy living, ranging from reimbursement for gym memberships to diet and nutrition counseling. The federal government is imposing penalties on hospitals and physicians, as well as providing financial incentives, all in an effort to keep patients well.

Yet, as men move into a stage of life where they are likely to have more time to devote to healthy living, research shows that they migrate to a more sedentary lifestyle (Matthews, Chen, Freedson, Buchowski, Beech, Pate, Troiano, 2008). So, what's wrong? Why is it so hard?

## Measures of Healthy Behavior and General Health Practices among 50+ Men

In 2015, an average of only 16% of males 45 and over met the federal 2008 Physical Activity Guidelines for Americans for aerobic activity and muscle strengthening, while 52% of that same cohort met neither set of guidelines (Health, United States, 2016). Worse, less than 3% of the country (men and women) live a healthy lifestyle, while other research suggests that over 90% of (all) American males rate themselves as possessing good, very good, or excellent health (Loprinzi, 2016)!

Other well-established measures further document men's health shortcomings. According to the Commonwealth Fund (Commonwealth Fund, 2000), men are out of touch when it comes to medical care. Their surveys found that 24% of men had not seen a physician during the prior year, three times the 8% rate for women. Moreover, 33% of men reportedly did not have a primary physician. In comparison, only 19% of women did not have a primary physician, with obstetrical or gynecological care only partially accounting for the difference. Finally, 24% of the men surveyed said that they would wait as long as possible before seeing a doctor, despite warning signs, with 17% of them indicating that they may wait at least a week!

## But We Started Out Okay

As I think about growing up in the 1960s and 70s and what influenced my life and the lives of my male friends, it is perplexing that men exhibit such unhealthy behavior at this stage of our lives. The drive and determination of our youth and early adulthood seems to have dissipated into indifference and neglect. As children and teens, boys work hard to make sports teams, learn to play instruments, become scouts, take up hobbies, prepare for college, or pursue part-time jobs. The sacrifices we made to enjoy our passions, what we valued at the time, taught us early on that sustained effort and commitment is a prerequisite for attaining our aspirations.

As young adults, men frequently make the connection between commitment and outcome when it comes to their families. They understand the importance of living in a good community, providing a college education for their children, and taking family vacations. They will sacrifice to provide these things for their loved ones. Ask any man who is putting in overtime, working late hours at the office, or traveling on business, what motivates him to press on and, without hesitation, many husbands and dads will pull out a photo of their wives and children.

Why it is that when we reach 50 years of age we have difficulty making this important connection between our health and the things most near and dear to our hearts? Are we simply out of gas? Has Mother Nature already inflicted too much on us? For some reason, when we reach the point in our lives when you'd think that life's clock would push us to double down on our health, the one most important factor that could extend our ability to enjoy life and leverage a return on all the investments we've made up to this point, we simply don't.

## Building the Case

I believe that there's reason for hope—hope that men of any age, but particularly men over 50, can rejuvenate their motivation for healthy living by leveraging the power of their values in the same fashion exhibited by the healthily-behaving men I studied. My belief in this pathway to health begins with a body of scientific and academic thought from the field of psychology that supports a psychologically and socially based approach to health. As I noted, motivation is a prerequisite for sustainable health, a point often overlooked and frequently glossed-over in the rush to meet a New Year's resolution, embark on the next fad diet, or purchase a gym membership. Through the data and stories in the pages to come I present the case that everyday men can adopt and sustain healthy behaviors, by first finding motivation through psychologically and socially based determinants and then designing a lifestyle based on this foundation.

My observations represent an alternative perspective to some commonly held approaches to developing a healthy lifestyle.

### 1. Cultural vs. Clinical

Clinical approaches have historically dominated healthcare. While certainly an important part of any effort to achieve good health, contemporary viewpoints give equal weight to social factors, witnessed by the conclusion that behavior represents the greatest influence on health. Cultural norms can influence behavior and a culture of health can, therefore, go a long way to improving health outcomes.

### 2. Internal vs. External

Extrinsic incentives are common in the promotion of health behaviors. Increasingly, behavioral economics, monetary rewards used to "jump-start" exercise and physical conditioning programs, seem to act as a means to drive behavior. Nevertheless, there is a substantial body of theory that suggests that such approaches can be short-lived, particularly if the rewards stop. My experience, and that of others who have studied this question even more extensively, suggests that an internal focus or intrinsic motivation is much more powerful and long lasting.

### 3. Social vs. Individual

Health behaviors, certainly in men, are traditionally seen as individually focused; it's *your* diet, *your* gym membership, *your* doctor's appointment, *your* progress in losing weight. The social approach stresses the social underpinnings of motivation: relationships, partnerships, and social activities, or, in its optimal form, the combination of social and physical activities.

### 4. Long-Term vs. Short-Term

By definition, your most valued relationships, the ones that generate the most emotion, are long-term in nature. Hence, they represent the most powerful of motivations. This perspective runs counter to the more common culture of health and fitness, which focuses on short-term success and measurement.

### 5. Ends vs. Means

The social approach is all about the endgame: graduations, weddings, and key life milestones as a source of motivation. Healthy behaviors are the necessary means to the achievement of the endgame. There is a plausible argument that a continual focus on these goals is the key to sustained, positive behavior.

As an executive, I always want to know what the experts think. Is my thinking and research consistent with theirs? How does it stand up? I'm not the first person to examine motivation, but I'm particularly interested in converting my work into actionable strategies that 50+ men and others can put into practice. In many ways, I'm a translator, so I want to know that my strategies are anchored in solid academic research, and, in particular, that there is ample and growing recognition that social factors and psychosocial determinants have a growing influence on the thinking on health behaviors.

So, before presenting these details and the strategies that follow, let's review the science of psychosocial motivation and examine the relationships between my results and the increasing recognition of the role of psychological and social factors in advancing health. Two factors anchor the argument that there is a strong relationship with a number of specific psychological theories offering support. The factors include: (1) the impact of behavior on health outcomes and, (2) psychosocial models of health (Ragin Fish, 2015).

## The Growing Recognition of Behavior in Health Outcomes

Medical experts agree that personal behavior is the most influential factor on one's health. Dr. Janet Corrigan of Dartmouth University reports the influence of healthy behaviors at 50%, while rating environment and genetics at 20% each and access to care at 10% (Corrigan, 2014). Dr. Jonathan Purtle at Drexel University's School of Public Health, citing 30 years of research and 10 studies, as published in the journal *Health Affairs*, rated behavior at 35% (Carrol-Scott, Henson, Kolker, Purtle, 2017). By any measure, behavior receives the highest rating.

Among the most glaring examples of the link between behavior and health, particularly in older adults, is diabetes (CDC, 2015). The US Center for Disease Control (CDC), through its National Center for Chronic Disease Prevention and Health Promotion, has declared diabetes an epidemic, with more than 29 million Americans living with diabetes and 86 million with prediabetes. 25% of those with diabetes don't know it and 90% of those with prediabetes are unaware (NCCD, 2016). The CDC's list of risk factors, which includes being overweight, 45 years or older, and being physically active less than 3 times a week (CDC, 2003) shows a connection between diabetes and behavior.

## Psychosocial Models of Health

Emotions can, and do, influence health behaviors. They are one of a number of psychological influences on health, which also include social support systems and personal traits. Sociological influences include familial, cultural, and community factors. Together, these factors (along with the inclusion of biological factors) form the bio-psychosocial models of well-being or a holistic health model (Ragin Fish, 2015). While health psychologists advance such concepts, their practical application increasingly appears in the medical community, in such practices as motivational interviewing. This recognition of the influence of emotional and social factors is consistent with the responses of the men I surveyed and interviewed. In both methodologies, the men cited emotional and social factors as inspirational sources for their behavior and, as noted earlier, incorporated these same factors in their diet and exercise practices.

While health psychologists have traced the relationship between health and emotions as far back as Hippocrates, and plotted the biological pathways through which this happens, my point here is more basic and foundational to the argument that motivation is an appropriate pathway to healthy behavior in 50+ men (Ragin Fish, 2015). That argument is simply that psychological and social factors are a valid source of motivation for healthy behavior in 50+ men.

## The Psychology of Behavior Change and Motivation

Academia considers my study to be a non-experimental design because I have not constructed a Randomized Controlled Trial (RCT) for comparison, nor have I attempted to manipulate variables in a highly structured fashion. I leave that to others. Rather, I consider my approach a teaching and learning-based methodology that seeks to identify models of behavior, by learning from those who exhibit the desired behavior. My theory and research are consistent with the research and the predominant theories in health psychology.

As a long-term executive, I am less interested in breaking new ground in scientific research and more focused on the practical needs of the targeted population. Documenting what works among a nation-wide sample of healthily-behaving men and uncovering the nuances of their lifestyles through in-depth interviews, creates a platform for the development of such models. The extents to which the men's responses reaffirm established health psychology bolster the case and the models emerge from this approach.

## A Mosaic of Psychology

There are a number of psychological theories and practices present in my findings, with varying degrees of application, a mosaic of psychology. Among the most dominant are: Positive Psychology, Mindfulness, Cognitive Behavior Theory (CBT), Message Framing, the recently published concept of Grit and, perhaps the most significant reference, Self-Determination Theory (SDT). I only touch briefly on each theory here. I provide references with more detail where the context of the discussion warrants them throughout the book. For now, my point is simply to present the theories to establish their place in the case to support a psychosocial approach to men's health and to substantiate the existence of each body of knowledge.

## Positive Psychology

Positive Psychology is a theory most frequently associated with Dr. Martin Seligman of the University of Pennsylvania, an early proponent of the clinical benefits of optimism. His insights and those of others represent a significant contribution to the understanding of behavior change and motivation. Aspects of Positive Psychology appear throughout the men's responses.

## Mindfulness

Mindfulness is a process often associated with meditation, with origins in Buddhism, brought to the Western world by Jon Kabat-Zinn. Contemporary definitions refer to it as "a state of being aware" and are associated with greater well-being and health (Branstrom, Duncan & Moskowitz, 2011). While meditation was not a dominant tactic exhibited by the men I studied, there is certainly a strong level of awareness between their values and behaviors.

## Cognitive Behavioral Theory/Therapy

University of Pennsylvania professor, psychiatrist Aaron T. Beck developed Cognitive Behavioral Therapy in the 1960s. CBT is a psychotherapy based on the cognitive model: the way that individuals perceive a situation (i.e., the way they see things) connects more closely to their reaction (i.e., the way that they behave) than the situation itself. The stories of the men, as well as the survey data, reflect the elements of CBT.

## Message Framing

Alexander Rothman and Peter Salovey have advanced the theory of message framing: health-relevant communications framed in terms of the benefits (gains) or costs (losses) associated with a particular behavior. Framing of such persuasive messages influences health decision-making (Rothman & Salovey, 1997). Messaging and the receptiveness of health-related messaging is an integral part of the dynamic in spurring motivation among 50+ men. I discuss the principles of message framing in Chapters 13, 14, and 15 in the discussions of men's health as heroism, women, and their health messaging to men and reshaping the cultural messaging of men's health respectively.

## Grit

Among the most recent concepts in psychology is a relatively new work by Professor Angela Duckworth, of the University of Pennsylvania, entitled "Grit". Relevant to men over 50 is Dr. Duckworth's conclusions that "we get grittier as we get older" and "you can grow grit from the inside out" (Duckworth, 2016). In fact, many of the men I spoke to told their own stories of grit and very much demonstrated their commitment to a gritty lifestyle.

## Self-Determination Theory

Some of psychology's most significant insights on motivation come from Edward L. Deci and Richard M. Ryan. In his book, *Drive*, Daniel Pink called them "the most influential behavioral scientists of their generation" (Pink, 2011).

In 1975, Deci published *Intrinsic Motivation*. In 2000, Ryan and Deci co-authored a seminal article in *American Psychologist*, which focused on self-motivation (Ryan & Deci, 2000), and in 2017 Ryan and Deci produced Self-Determination Theory, a systematic review of the theory.

The 2000 article outlines Self-Determination Theory (SDT) as anchored by their belief that intrinsic or internal motivations are far superior to extrinsic or external motivations, particularly in maintaining the desired behavior over the long-term. According to Ryan and Deci, the production of intrinsic motivations takes place when one meets the three key supportive psychological needs: autonomy, relatedness, and competence. They characterize autonomy as the ability of individuals to make choices about their behavior without outside influences. Relatedness concerns behaviors that create some form of attachment and security with others. Competence is the ability to carry out the behavior or improve your mastery of the desired behaviors.

While Ryan and Deci clearly advocate for the superiority of intrinsic or internal motivations, they offer another pathway to sustainable behavior, emanating from extrinsic or outside motivations: what they call identification and integration. Identification occurs when individuals consciously value a behavior and accept it as their own because of its importance to themselves. Integration is the full assimilation with or the coming together of one's values and needs (Ryan & Deci, 1985).

Summarizing the findings of Ryan, Deci, and other SDT researchers in a 2007 article in *Men's Health*, Tom McGrath wrote, "The more self-determined we are—that is the more we're doing what we want to do and aren't being forced to do—the happier and more successful we tend to be." (McGrath, 2007).

McGrath provides an example of self-identified motivation in Dr. Phillip Wilson, a psychologist and former pro soccer player, upon reflecting on his time in the gym: "Quite frankly, it hurts but I do it because I value the health benefits." (McGrath, 2007).

The research of Ryan and Deci is significant because it demonstrates that the values and priorities of our 50+ men can indeed serve as a source of intrinsic motivation for healthy behavior, either directly or through the extrinsic motivational pathways, and become a sustaining force for healthy living.

Collectively, this body of psychology represents some of the most foundational theory in the field and related therapies in psychiatry. These theories affirm the responses of my research participants and create a platform to develop a model to represent the characteristics exhibited by the healthily behaving men.

## The Harvard Study of Adult Development

While not a psychological theory, there is one final reference in the study of behavior, and specifically the link between social determinants and health in men, that warrants inclusion in this review: the Harvard Study of Adult Development, one of the most comprehensive longitudinal studies in history. For over 75 years, researchers have tracked the lives of 724 men and examined the factors that influence their health. According to its director, Dr. Robert Waldinger, "the clearest message that we get from this study is that good relationships keep us happier and healthier" and that "social connections are really good for us." (Waldinger, 2015).

As perhaps the most significant study of men and the health impacts of social factors, it speaks volumes and further validates to the social pathway to health in men.

## Male Cognitive Behavioral Alignment (MCBA)

The men I studied connected the dots between their life's priorities and their health behaviors. The association is strong enough to trigger action. They don't simply think about how healthy behavior *could* enhance their emotional priorities and personal values, they act on them. This is distinguishing and significant.

Drilling deeper through their stories, I learned that the men often seize the opportunity to accomplish multiple goals when carrying out their behaviors. By walking with their wives or sharing a healthy meal with a friend, the men were able to advance their social objectives simultaneously with their health-related practices. I call this the Male Cognitive Behavioral Alignment (MCBA) Model. This is a two-tiered model that includes: (1) awareness of the value-behavior relationship (i.e., men recognize the link between the achievement of their life's priorities and their health), and (2) the integration of these priorities into their diet and exercise practices (i.e., men walk or share healthy meals with their wives). Men achieving this state of psychological, social, and behavioral alignment help themselves sustain their behaviors.

## Cycle of Healthy Behavior (CHB)

I learned that when men initiate healthy behavior, because of these perceptual associations, their actions produce a biological reaction and they feel good! This good feeling spurs the motivation to continue the behavior, creating what I call the Cycle of Healthy Behavior (CHB), the perpetuation of the behavior consistent with the biopsychosocial models in the literature.

## Lifestyle Architecture

The men who exhibit Male Cognitive Behavior Alignment and the Cycle of Healthy Behavior do so within the structure of their own personal behavior. This framework contains a number of lower-order, but still very important, functional motivators (what I later call micro-motivators), proactive social activities, and other forward-looking motivating events that add to and operationalize their dominant life priorities. I call this their Lifestyle Architecture: the strategies, tactics, routines, and rituals that make up their healthy living toolbox, which in turn creates a personalized behavioral structure representing the engine fueled by the MCBA to propel the men into the Cycle of Health. I found instances where the Lifestyle Architecture of some men is so sophisticated, they maintain elaborate contingency plans and options designed to stand up to the inevitable roadblocks to healthy behaviors that life brings. Together, Male Cognitive Behavior Alignment, the Cycle of Health, and an overarching Lifestyle Architecture represent the pathway to health, as displayed by the healthily-behaving men.

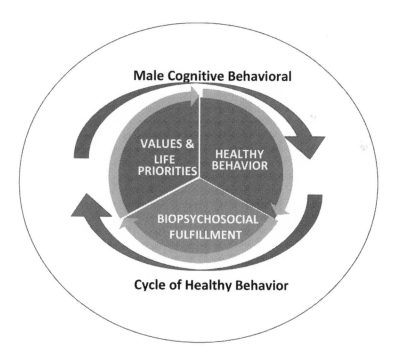

Figure 1: MCBA Cycle

## The Psychology Applied

I had the benefit of knowing a long-time primary care physician for a few years during the twilight of his medical career and, ultimately, his life. He was my father-in-law, Dr. Frank Iula, and he personified the traditional primary care doctor. He understood motivation and used his understanding of his patients' lives to assure compliance to their clinical needs. He lived in the community, and—if he didn't know the patient from town—he made sure to ask about their lives, interests, and families during their appointments. Further, he would make notes on the oversized index cards he used for his patients' medical histories and to chronicle their important life events. As a regular practice, he would refer to these personal notes and update them as he saw his patients over the years. This was his manual version of what we now call an Electronic Medical Record (EMR), and his personal notes about patients today would go in an electronic "field" with a designation of "social risk" or the like. There was an endless line of patients at his funeral, many of whom cherished him and would never think of ignoring his medical instructions. In the absence of a well-defined body of knowledge or medical instruction that taught him to perform what we now called "motivational interviewing," he intuitively understood the value of knowing his patients and the importance of leveraging that knowledge to better their health outcomes. He intuitively understood the psychology of health care. Yes, what's old is new, indeed.

Today, American medicine is embracing Dr. Iula's approach. More than ever, health care providers adopt the form of health behavioral counseling called Motivational Interviewing (MI), which seeks to tie patient health decisions to long-term, specific goals through provider-based education and dialog (White, Gazewood, & Mounsey, 2007). Martins and McNeil (2009) found motivational interviewing to be beneficial in the treatment of a host of physical health issues, by helping encourage lifestyle changes and adherence to treatment. Specifically, patients at risk of diet- and exercise-related health complications, treated with MI alone or in combination with other interventions, reported increased self-efficacy related to diet and exercise, increased physical activity, reduced caloric intake, increased fruit and vegetable consumption, and decreased body-mass-index scores. Diabetic patients experienced similar results, in addition to better control of glucose levels. Additionally, MI even appeared to help patients improve their oral hygiene.

In other words, as basic as it may sound, health care providers are increasingly focusing on the connection between clinical success and the personal, social, and emotional aspirations of their patients. They are asking them about their interests in life and linking these goals to their medical care plans, as a way to increase adherence. Therefore, when a grandpa tells his doctor that he wants to dance at his grand-daughter's wedding, the physician can use this goal to motivate grandpa to follow doctor's orders, fill his prescription, and make sure he schedules a follow-up visit. The practice is fairly simple on the surface, but represents a big change for the medical community mind-set.

## The Closing Argument

So, why study motivation in 50+ men? The case is clear: it starts with a burning platform for change, the poor state of men's health, the growth of behavior-influenced chronic disease, and an ominous male-mortality rate. It continues with the understanding that the most important influence on our health is our own behavior.

Steve, from our New Jersey focus group, understood that healthy living is a means to an end and a pathway to the achievement of his priorities in life. He was so far down this path that he couldn't see why not everyone saw the connection between healthy living and its benefits. We should all aspire to be in Steve's place.

# 2

## Cracking the Code: Motivation in 50+ Men

ALAN DOES YOGA AND enjoys healthy meals with his wife. David runs 5-K races with his daughter. Vijay walks the halls of a shopping mall. Jay enjoys eating salmon dinners with is his friend. Carmen regularly walks the high school track, splitting time between a buddy and his wife. Bob swims at the YMCA, where he watches his granddaughter compete. Day after day, week after week, and year after year, these men live healthy lives. They don't participate in triathlons or extreme sports.

By comparison to the extreme athletes, their routines are rather modest, tailored to their life circumstances. To advance their life's priorities and leverage the maximum benefit from their time invested, the men frequently fit their health behaviors in with their social interests. Consistent and varied, they plan for contingencies and keep active in numerous ways.

What's extraordinary about the men I interviewed is their shared experiences: all are over 50, all willingly adopted their lifestyle, none received compensation for their activities, and their doctors did not inspire their behavior. Not one attributed their behavior to the shoes they wear or the size of their gym, a pill, dietary supplement, special diet, or exercise equipment. No, they simply love their active lifestyle and the benefits that result from it, including the ability to keep up with the grandchildren, quality time with a spouse or significant other, travel, employment, community activities, and the like.

For them, health is a means to an end, and the endgame is the advancement of their life priorities, which are always at the top of their minds. In short, these men exhibit Male Cognitive Behavioral Alignment. They maintain conscious awareness between the achievement of their most valued priorities and their health. What I heard from Alan, David, Vijay, Carmen, and Bob, and most of the men I interviewed, echoes the results of my nationwide survey. Men over 50 can indeed lead a healthy lifestyle and sustain healthy behaviors. By studying their lifestyle architecture, men can construct a new model for their health, a psychosocial or social model with broad applications.

My obsession, what I sought-out to do, is to understand the motivation of healthily behaving men over 50, the source of their motivation, the beliefs that shape this motivation, and their day-to-day practices.

I believe that the state of men's health is such that it requires a new model, one that dives deeper into the core of a man's belief system and taps that inner strength needed to overcome the traditional barriers to behavior change. As internal emotional factors can and do regulate and motivate healthily-behaving 50+ men in a positive way, then why not design a lifestyle based on this foundation? If behavior is the biggest influence on our health, do we crack the code of sustainable health if we understand what controls behavior and design a model based on those factors?

Doing so could open the floodgates to a world of benefits that range from longer and more enjoyable and fulfilling lives to reductions in health care costs, improved clinical outcomes, and intangible benefits like the memories of grandchildren—no small thing when you are talking about 50 million of us!

## A Model Designed for Men, Designed by Men

To get the answers to my questions and find the secret sauce of motivation for healthy living among 50+ men, I went to the best source, the ultimate experts: men 50 and over who live healthily. As a 50+ man, I understand the skepticism of our age group. Products and strategies that claim to improve our health inundate us. With this in mind, I wanted to take an approach that I could honestly say uses the practices and perspective of men like us: men who've shared our experiences, know the challenges of behavior change firsthand, and represent a true picture of what healthy behavior really looks like. I wanted credibility.

I also wanted more than statistics. Yes, I sought the power of a national survey, but I also wanted to know how healthy living works on a human level. I wanted stories of men who maintain their behavior in a real-world context. With this in mind, I set out on a three-phased process to see what I could learn from the men: one quantitative and two qualitative. I prescreened the men involved in the study and determined that they maintained healthy behaviors that reduce health risks such as heart disease, diabetes, and colorectal cancer, as established by Dr. Nash (Institute of Medicine, 2001).

The research for this book represents a personal mission for me and a tribute to the men who were willing to share their experiences and feelings. There are no sponsors or grants. I personally funded all elements of the research myself, including the nationwide survey, five focus groups, and the interviews. I engaged marketing specialists and student researchers to support the project team and designed the survey questionnaires. The references to medical experts and behavioral scientists are products of my interviews and the conclusions that I've drawn resulting from this work.

My first research phase was a nationwide survey of 1,000 men. The survey had four principal objectives: (1) to develop a profile of healthily living 50+ men, (2) to identify the major life priorities of these men, (3) to determine if life priorities are a source of motivation, and (4) to solicit opinions which would guide my thinking about the broader applications to the contemporary state of men's health.

The second research phase included two focus groups, each comprised of eight to ten men, one in New Jersey, and one in San Francisco. New Jersey and California nationally rank high in the number of healthy residents. The groups served two purposes: to prescreen questions for the survey, and to provide stories, personal accounts, illustrations, and examples, that added an incredibly personal and descriptive level of meaning that was both enlightening, in terms of the research, and personally inspirational.

Even more significant was the third phase: personal interviews. I spoke to 20 men about their motivation for healthy living and the ways in which they maintain their behavior and supplemented the interviews with a group session, comprised of 13 of the original 20. Together, the focus groups and the interviews humanize the survey data, demonstrate how men have confronted life's struggles, and found motivation for healthy living in that which is most important to them. Their stories offer lessons, which I share throughout the book and incorporate into my motivational blueprint for healthy living. Let's start by looking at the survey results of what 1,000 healthily living men can tell us about their motivation to live healthily.

## What Do the Men Consider Most Important for Healthy Living?

What does healthy behavior look like in a 50+ man? What are the attributes that these men exhibit? What do they consider as their most important behaviors? What habits, routines, and rituals do they employ to maintain their behavior? Is optimism relevant? What do they see as the benefits of a healthy lifestyle? Here's what the men had to say.

### Attributes

50+ men with healthy behavior exhibit a number of key attributes:

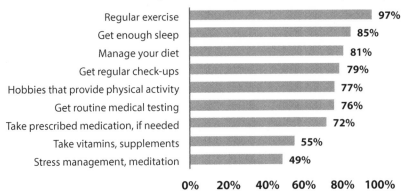

Figure 2: Important Attributes For A Healthy Lifestyle

## Habits, Routines, and Rituals

How do the men turn their motivation into a long-term sustainable commitment? My findings indicate that the men rely heavily on habits, routines, and rituals: what I call the guardrails of healthy behavior.

So, what are these healthy habits? You'll see that they represent the next level of commitment, a granular operationalization of the broader motivating factors cited previously that are an integral part of their daily living. The men responded as follows:

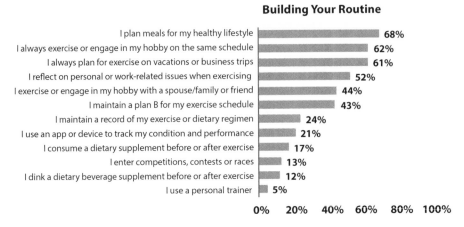

Figure 3: Building Your Routine

## The Value of Optimism

There are many who believe that optimism is important to shape and maintain successful behaviors, so I measured the level of optimism among the participants and solicited their thoughts on the subject. Here's what I found:

- 60% indicated that they considered themselves either very or extremely optimistic.

- 75% indicated that optimism was an important factor in maintaining a healthy lifestyle.

The importance of optimism held across all ages categories:

- 61% of men aged 70 and over considered themselves optimistic.

- 58% of men 60-69 considered themselves optimistic.

- 62% of men 50-59 considered themselves optimistic.

## Benefits of a Healthy Lifestyle

Expectations and purpose are measures of motivation. They provide insight into the endgame and add to a deeper understanding of the "why" of healthy living. Accordingly, I asked the men what they saw as the benefits of their healthy behavior. They had no trouble giving me plenty of examples that they perceive as tangible benefits of their effort to live healthily. As you will see in the section to come, the benefits responses tie directly to the motivation responses and reinforce the notion that life priorities are a principal source of inspiration for a healthy lifestyle. Here are the men's top-ranked benefits.

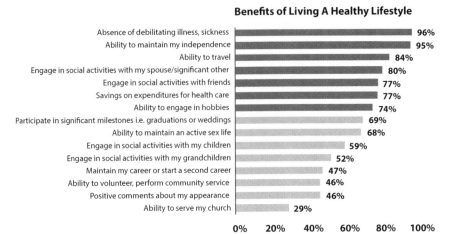

Figure 4: Benefits of Living A Healthy Lifestyle

There's a management strategy known as backward reasoning. It suggests that one way to go about achieving a goal is to have a clear picture of what success looks like from which you (or a team) can work backwards to determine what it would take to achieve that goal. While I'm always hesitant to use a word like backwards in promoting positive, forward-looking behavior, in this instance, I believe it works.

To live healthily, a man needs to know exactly what that means and what he can reasonably expect. With the media bombarding 50+ men with messages targeting multiple demographics, defining a model that specifically applies to them is critical, and illustrations can go a long way to promoting clarity and understanding. Applying backward reasoning, 50+ men can study the profile of the healthily-behaving men from my survey and begin really to understand the fundamentals of this behavior—what it is, what it looks like, and its benefits.

Kevin provides a great illustration of the 50+ healthy-man profile. He embeds exercise and diet into his lifestyle and a year-round diversified schedule of activity, where he involves his still young children, that enables him to carry the healthy behaviors he adapted as a young man into his 50s. Still playing competitive sports, he's developed supportive partnerships through his teammates that fuel his own competitive fires and promote the discipline he says is essential to his healthy habits. He sees his priorities in life as a combination of factors, which he thinks about a lot, and exerts a strong influence on his life. "It's like a combination—of my family, my career, my faith, and my health. I think they're all important."

Besides a longer life, Kevin believes that his healthy lifestyle has other benefits: "It clears the mind, helps you think better, so you make better decisions in your life—you have more energy; you feel better."

With a better idea of exactly what it means to live healthily, let's now turn to what the men value most, their top priorities, and extend our understanding of this new approach to men's health.

## What Men Value Most: The Top Priorities

So, what are the life priorities that shape a man's beliefs and potentially his behavior? How do the respective priorities rank? Do men's priorities change as they age? For answers, I asked the men to identify their priorities and rate their importance. The answers add further dimension to our understanding of a man's beliefs.

## Top Priority: Spouses/Significant Others

When it comes to their life's priorities, the men are very clear, providing consistent answers in response to various forms of questioning. The following chart shows that the highest priority in all age groups across the board is spending time with spouse, partner, or significant other. The percentages adjust for age as seen below, for example job/career reduces in importance as the men reach retirement age.

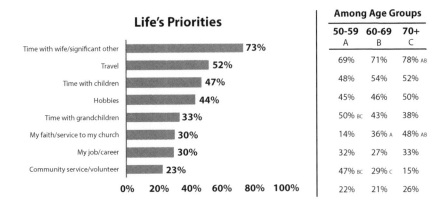

| | Among Age Groups | | |
| --- | :---: | :---: | :---: |
| | **50-59** | **60-69** | **70+** |
| | A | B | C |
| Time with wife/significant other — 73% | 69% | 71% | 78% AB |
| Travel — 52% | 48% | 54% | 52% |
| Time with children — 47% | 45% | 46% | 50% |
| Hobbies — 44% | | | |
| Time with grandchildren — 33% | 50% BC | 43% | 38% |
| My faith/service to my church — 30% | 14% | 36% A | 48% AB |
| My job/career — 30% | 32% | 27% | 33% |
| Community service/volunteer — 23% | 47% BC | 29% C | 15% |
| | 22% | 21% | 26% |

Figure 5: Life's Priorities

## The Importance of the Spouse/Significant Other Grows with Age

As men age they increasingly value time with their wives or significant others.

- 69% of men 50-59 rated "spending time with their spouse or significant other" as their number one life priority. This number grows to 71% among men 60-69 and 78 % in the 70+ age group.

- Travel increases slightly between the 50-59 and 60-69 age brackets, moving from 48 % to 54% respectively, but then decreasing to 52 % in the 70+ group.

- Hobbies are at a high of 50% in the 50-59 age group, but then drop to just 38 % in importance in the 70+ group.

- As one might guess, "time with grandchildren" grows significantly from 14 % in the 50s age range to 36% in their 60s and ultimately 48 % among those 70 and older.

- The opposite occurs with "My job/career," which starts with a priority ranking of 47 % among those 50-59, but then drops to 29 % in the 60-69 group and then to 15% in the 70+ group.

## Marital Status or a Significant Other Makes a Difference

Marital status or the presence of a significant other in the lives of the men makes a significant difference in their priorities. When compared to the responses of single men or those that are divorced, widowed, or separated, the married men place greater importance on their personal relationships, children, and grandchildren. Less impacted priorities by marital status or a personal relationship include hobbies, community service, and jobs/careers.

## Priorities: A Source of Motivation?

Can the social, emotional, and personal priorities in a man's life serve as a source of motivation for healthy living? The men I asked overwhelmingly said, "Yes." When compared to other possible motivators for healthy behavior, such as a physician's advice or financial incentives from a health insurer, personal priorities ranked considerably higher with more than three-quarters of the men I surveyed, indicating that priorities play a major role in providing them motivation. The youngest of the age groups, those 50-59, produced the highest rating for the influence of priorities on healthy behaviors, suggesting that men recognize the importance of these factors early on as they age. Nevertheless, priorities dominated all the age categories, demonstrating the sustainability of priorities as a motivator among these men.

Rod personifies a man with an active lifestyle grounded in his life's priorities: his wife, his grandchildren, and his brother. When interviewed, he proudly tells me that he has maintained the same size clothes for decades, a measure of commitment to his behavior. Rod's response to my question about priorities is consistent with the survey data on priorities and motivations:

Well, I'd like to—I'd like to stay healthy. I'd like to stay active. I'd like to be able to stay around as long as I can, you know. I think I would like to make sure that my quality of life and the people that are in my—you know; in my life—I don't want to be a burden to anyone. I think that it's—it's my—my goal is to—to have a good quality of life and not burden somebody—burden anyone with having to watch me deteriorate or suffer, and so on and so forth. So, does that keep me healthy or does that give me motivation to try to keep doing things and—yes.

## Men Frequently Think About Their Priorities

Strengthening the association between social priorities and motivation is the frequency with which the healthily living men think about their priorities, a core element of their cognitive alignment. Almost three-quarters of my study participants said they think about their priorities once a week or more.

## Motivation: The Sources

What are the specific factors that drive motivation? How anchored are they in a man's emotional and social relationships? Do they represent a pathway to creating a new psychosocial model of men's health? My discussion of the perceived benefits of a healthy lifestyle gave you a preview. Now let's look at the results when asked the question directly.

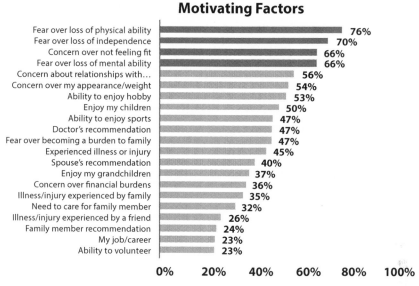

Figure 6: Motivating Factors

## Fear

Fear over the loss of physical and mental ability and the loss of independence is the most significant motivator of healthy behavior, according to my survey. Other factors such as relationships, children, the inability to play sports, and illness and injury are significant, but somewhat less motivating.

Losing the ability to function independently is a scary thought. You would think that anyone who considered the implications for themselves, let alone their families, would be scared straight to the gym and the fruit and vegetable aisle at the supermarket. Unfortunately, this is not always the case; however, our study participants suggest that a dose of reality goes a long way.

Among those surveyed, fear over loss of physical and/or mental ability and independence, were the top two motivating factors for both starting and maintaining a healthy lifestyle. Although certainly no one wants to lose their ability to function or their independence, in the survey findings, we will see a strong tie to other highly rated motivators. When viewed in this context, we see that what motivates our men are very specific and tangible factors that they value.

These factors explain why fear, as expressed by our participants, is more than just a concern over their personal well-being, but also encompass a more complex and comprehensive set of values that drive their motivation. Other factors such as relationships, children, and inability to play sports, illness, and injury are strong, but somewhat less motivating, than fear, but represent related factors.

Beyond fear, the next tier of motivating factors provides further insight into what inspires healthily living men. In many ways, they reflect the "at risk" factors if a man suffered the loss of his physical or mental capacities, an approach often seen in advertisements targeted to this population.

As a group, the ratings of this second tier of motivators ranged from a low of 45% (experienced illness or injury) to a high of 56% (concern about my relationship with my spouse or significant other). Of the eight factors in this tier, four of the factors were in the 50th percentile and are largely diverse. I've already noted that the top-rated factor from the men is concern about their relationship with their spouse or partner. The high rating for concern about the spouse/significant other is consistent with other ratings of life priorities.

Tim exhibits a common theme seen in many of the men, a direct line of motivation stemming from a strong awareness of what's important in his life. When we spoke, he described a period in his life when he smoked cigarettes and would get drunk on weekends. I asked him when his healthy behavior kicked-in. His response spoke volumes:

> It was like an epiphany. I guess it was, like—well, my youngest was born. It was after she was born in August, and then in September when my 16-year-old daughter's birthday was coming up, and she was like, "Dad, you know you, you got to stop smoking. You're not going to be able to walk me down

the aisle for my wedding." My mother had just quit, so I said, "All right, I'll do it." And, I just did it. Yes, it was very difficult, but it's been nine years. It's funny, because the older kids remember that I smoked and she (the youngest) doesn't.

## Implications for the Constituencies of Men's Health

My primary objective is to serve 50+ men. They need to find a source of motivation for healthy living, improve their behaviors, and reverse the horrible state of their health. And—fast! That said, the data and the insights offered in my survey send a strong message to the wives, partners, and individuals who love them. Further, there are implications for stakeholders in the world of health care, what I call the three Ps-providers, payers (i.e., health insurers), and policy makers. In the later chapters, I will speak more directly to these constituencies and outline some very specific proposals that address the broader context of men's health in our world today. Here is one example pulled from the survey, one that I briefly touched on earlier in my story about Dr. Iula.

## Men and Their Physicians

More men need to speak to their doctors about their priorities. Of the men surveyed, only 32% indicated that they discussed their personal priorities with their physicians. Not a hugely significant number, but not surprising given the current state of American health care. What is significant is that:

- 81% of the men who discussed priorities with their doctor indicated that these conversations worked well.

Breaking down the numbers among age brackets, men between 50 and 59 are more likely to have spoken with their physician about their life's priorities.

- 37% spoke with their physicians compared to 31% among those between 60 and 69, and 27% among those 70 and above.

From the other side, the findings suggest that it would serve physicians to initiate a non-clinical, more in-depth conversation (e.g., conduct motivational interviewing) with men about their life priorities. The lesson for both physicians and their 50+ male patients is to communicate! Not just the superficial stuff, but a conversation that touches on what's most important to these men, and, more directly, what's most likely to stimulate positive health behavior: their wives or significant others, children, grandchildren, or whatever they signal is a priority. Yes, it's tough in a short visit, but it could yield valuable benefits, and such benefits could end up reducing costs and improving clinical outcomes, music to the ears of the insurers and policy makers.

## Lessons from the Men

Healthily-behaving men over 50 have very distinctive and consistent lifestyles. Their practices, priorities, and motivations form a model aligned with the leading theories in psychology, particularly those based on the emotional and social influences on health. Let's review the most significant findings, those that form the foundation of this new approach to men's health.

## Hope

In a word, what our healthy men have provided through this survey is hope. Hope for the thousands and thousands of American 50+ men who struggle with their health. Unable to latch on and sustain a healthy lifestyle, their unhealthy behavior has put them at risk in a very serious way. The numbers don't lie. Beyond the very real clinical risks are the social, emotional, and personal risks of not experiencing everything that life has to offer: time with their wives or partners, travel, milestones in the lives of their children and grandchildren, second careers, hobbies, and the like. Hope gives us purpose and it inspires us like no other.

The lesson is simple. Your motivation is right in front of you and it can form a pathway to healthy behavior. For some reason, we just don't see it. Perhaps, as men, we have that caveman belief that we're invincible. We're not. Maybe we take things for granted. We shouldn't. Whatever the reasons or the mindset or the circumstances, let's learn from this study. Allow yourself to be coachable and open your minds to the instruction and wisdom found in their responses.

In the chapters that follow, I build on my own story and the lessons from the men and present a 10-step motivational blueprint for healthy behavior, one based on a social platform that's more about shaping and inspiring behavior than any particular diet or exercise program. It is simple, straightforward, and easy to adopt. Instructions included! In addition, with a newfound source of motivation and your behavioral guardrails in place, you'll dramatically increase the chances that your gym membership won't lapse, you'll stick to the diet, and you'll begin to enjoy your healthy lifestyle, as you see the positive impact on the achievement of your life's priorities. Follow me. The journey begins.

# 3

## My Motivation

JOHN SHEETS IS AN 80-year old Army and Coast Guard Reserve veteran and competitive weight lifter who bench presses 5 days a week when he's in competition. A USA powerlifting gold medal winner, John has set a number of records (Nark, 2016). George Siedel is 72 and a professor at the University of Michigan. According to the *Wall Street Journal*, Siedel is a disciple of a Chinese practice called qigong, based on gentle movements, meditation, and breathing. He supplements his qigong with Tai Chi, has a fitness center membership, and every other day does strength training (Murphy, 2017). These men are extraordinary, motivated, and committed. Their stories are fascinating and proof that men over 50 are capable of living healthily and remaining active as they age. Nevertheless, they are outliers, representing only a small percent of the men over 50.

While I applaud their accomplishments and feel inspired when I see any man over 50 bucking the trend, I also recognize that a cultural shift of the magnitude I'm advocating requires a broad-based movement. There will always be exceptional individuals. My focus is the Everyman: those who struggle to adopt healthy behavior, and for whom a bike ride, a walk, or a light swim on a consistent basis would represent real progress. These men need motivation, structure, and support to adopt and sustain a healthy lifestyle. I want to help the Everyman in us all.

My own experience, in large measure, fuels my passion. Now 63, I've witnessed first-hand how exercise can serve as an antidote to the stress and adversity life brings. Initially finding exercise as a defense mechanism to combat life's battles, I've grown to appreciate the benefits of diet and exercise, discovering how it can help you look, feel, and sleep better. For me, these benefits create an urge to be socially active, seek out fun, and remain competitive professionally—things I've come to appreciate increasingly with age.

Motivation for my lifestyle originally came from my most cherished and valued priorities and was in large measure influenced through a decade as a single dad—although, more contemporarily, because I really enjoy it.

Like Sheets and Siedel, I relish the products of my behavior and I'm able to meet Dr. Nash's criteria for a healthy lifestyle. Unlike Sheets and Siedel, my routine is not quite so exotic; I don't power lift or rely on Eastern rites, nor do I run marathons, compete in triathlons, or undertake mountain climbing. My approach centers on consistency and the practicality of a man whose routine revolves around full-time employment, a reasonable diet, cardio workouts, strength training, and a strong dose of stretching. Intertwined and driving this behavior is an active life, socially and professionally, Male Cognitive Behavioral Alignment or what I sometimes like to alternatively call the Everyman's Life Style.

Where did this all start? Why did I find sanctuary in healthy behavior? It's hard to say. I've often thought that it might be a product of my upbringing. In the 60s and 70s, my mother was an early entrant into the women's fitness craze with the leotards and the exercise bike in the basement. Dad played softball and some basketball, carrying his youthful pursuits well into his 40s and 50s.

As a youth, I played sports and was active year-round. In college, I maintained a level of activity through intramural sports. As I entered my senior year, with my parent's divorce looming and the prospect of embarking on the next phase of my life, I began what would turn into a lifelong passion for running.

Setting out to make my way in the world as a 20-something man, I continued what came naturally. I ran, played softball, and generally stayed active without a whole lot of attention to diet. After all, I was in my twenties and burned-off whatever I ate. What I didn't know was that I was about to embark on a series of events over the next 30-plus years that would be extremely stressful, disrupt my goals, and require a major adjustment in the course I had plotted. Aided in no small part by healthy practices, as I look back today, I'm extremely happy with where I am in life and the perspective that I gained through the adversity. What began as my coping mechanism migrated into a passion, and, for that, I'm grateful.

As men, a number of factors influence our lives. We have the opportunity, no matter what age, to learn and adopt new ideas, especially those that can be positive and life changing. Regardless of your path, it's important to know that you can mold and shape your life to meet your needs and circumstances. You may find relevance in my pathway. It may spur ideas and inspiration in your life. Either way, at minimum, I hope my story triggers thoughts on how you might craft your own lifestyle architecture and enjoy the benefits. In my case, the most meaningful factors in the 40-plus years of my journey fall into three categories: marriage, children, and career. Here is a glimpse of the events that shaped the course of my life and resulted in the passion I hold today for healthy behavior and the state of all men over 50.

## Marriage

I've been married for almost 10 years. Her name is Maria. She is the love of my life and my children and grandson love her. Life is good, and she both shares and supports my healthy behavior. Maria has taken me to a whole other level in terms of diet and nutrition. We share a mutual interest in continuous learning and longevity. Our life together has become a major source of motivation for living healthy. Travel, planning family events, and home improvements are just a few of the items that provide a robust agenda year-round that keeps me at the gym and thinking healthily. I want to enjoy all that life has to offer. Maria exemplifies the value of partnerships and the impact of women on men's health, two topics I cover later in the book. She's wife number three.

My first marriage gave me two wonderful sons and later a grandson. For that, I am ever grateful. It also produced a high level of stress that literally had me wearing a path on the running trail. One story in particular illustrates the adversity that I confronted in my 20s.

Not long into the marriage, we became pregnant. Early one evening, I was just home from work when I received a call from the nurse at my wife's doctor's office. She had just finished a routine visit in the last month of the pregnancy—seems the doctor couldn't hear the baby's heartbeat. My wife was distraught. The nurse was preparing me for what I would shortly encounter.

Tests confirmed the doctor's suspicions. The baby had died, strangled by its umbilical cord. The doctor would have to deliver the stillborn. As I watched my wife give birth to what turned out to be our baby boy, the expression on his face carved an impression that will forever stay etched in my mind. To manage the heartache, I found myself running and exercising. It eased some of the pain and gave me the comfort I needed to support my wife. Eventually, the clarity of thought and peacefulness produced by the workouts enabled me to move forward. I felt good when I ran, and it went a long way to coping with that image.

Fortunately, over the next decade, we went on to have two healthy boys. Unfortunately, the marriage didn't last. With joint custody, I saw the boys on the weekends and made it a point to have dinner with them every Wednesday night. Socially, I became involved with a woman I met through work. We dated and, after about five years, I married again. For reasons beyond both of us, and most unfortunate, the marriage was short-lived. Again, I found myself turning to exercise as the remedy to navigate through yet another transition.

## Children

If there's anything that provides motivation in your life, it's your children. They say a parent will do almost anything for their kids. And, it is true. As my life unfolded, I found myself in the position of being a single dad in my early 40s. Post marriage one and with a short overlap with marriage two, the boys were living with me full-time. My oldest was in seventh grade, my younger son in second. It was a labor of love but a challenge nonetheless. Back-to-school nights, packing lunches, homework, and school sports consumed my world, which I also had to juggle with my job. Overall, it was tough, but we made it work as a family. Parenthood, particularly at the level of engagement I was at, has a way of putting life in perspective. When your son gets sick all over you in a crowded movie theater; or you get a call at work from the school nurse that you boy's faucet-like bloody nose has erupted again, you deal with it. When you hear that the wheel of your teenage son's car almost came off on a major highway as he returned home from a trip to visit his girlfriend, again, you deal with it. As all parents know, you handle it swiftly and responsively, but you take it in stride, knowing that it's all part of being a parent. Yes, suddenly, the small stuff seems so insignificant, and you focus like a laser on the big picture and the long-term.

For me, this included the desire to keep up with the boys, earn a living that would provide a secure future, and generally tend to their needs. It was clear that I needed strength and stamina for the long haul, and that I'd better pay attention to my health to ensure that they were always all right. The connection worked. I bought some exercise equipment for the basement, kept running, and began to enter 5K races. My routine increased as they grew up, and I had the time to do things like run in the morning before work.

Two of my most memorable experiences as a single dad came in 1999 and 2007 respectively, when my sons were high school seniors. In each of those years, I volunteered our home for a PTA fundraiser, the Holiday House Tour, a very nice event where local residents decorate their homes for the holidays and open them up for people to tour. It was my own personal statement to myself; I was able to validate our standing as a family, albeit without a female lead, and show the community that we could give back to the schools.

In 1999, I wasn't dating anyone at the time, so the women of the PTA were a big help. They provided decorating tips and guided me to deals on carpets and furniture to dress up the house. I went all out. On top of that, they arranged for a florist to transform our dining room into a winter wonderland. Among his touches were the placement of 100 roses in a Christmas tree my landscaper had donated. In the PTA's promotional material, they advertised our home as "The Men's Home," featuring with my collection of sports bobble head dolls in lieu of the more traditional display of cultured figurines on display at the other homes. It was a wonderful and proud moment for the boys and me.

In 2007, my younger son was a senior, so I again volunteered my home for the tour. By that time, I had met Maria. She was a big help in what was, by then, a significantly renovated house—another proud moment as people from all over town came through our impeccably decorated home.

As a benchmark, the tours proved a great measuring stick that gave me the impetus to continue striving for success in all facets of my life. Diet and exercise had become my secret weapon in my life's battles, and the house tours were symbolic of my victory over what life had thrown at me.

## Career

As an undergraduate, I developed an interest in political science and eventually earned a master's degree in public policy. While in graduate school, I met a colleague who was a bartender at the time but had political ambitions. The colleague left the program but went on to become a congressional aide and was eventually elected to a seat on the board that runs the county government. In New Jersey, we call them freeholders.

When I completed graduate school, we reconnected and he offered me a position as a Deputy County Administrator. I jumped at the opportunity. It was a dream job. I was fresh out of school, my head packed with ideas about public management and a welcoming official who sought good government. It set me on a career path that was rewarding and fulfilling, and never dull.

The master's degree also provided an entrée into the academic world. I quickly learned that I could earn a few extra bucks and enhance my resume by teaching as an adjunct professor. I went for it, teaching evening courses at the community college and nearby universities, ultimately teaching graduate courses in the same public policy program from which I graduated. Today, some 40 years later, I'm still teaching public policy. It's a devotion, one that keeps me sharp and continuously learning.

Professionally, I went on to take the top administrative post in a municipal government, then returned to the county as county administrator. At 32, I was the chief administrative official, a highly visible position in a county of a half-million residents, overseeing upwards of 3,000 employees and a budget that exceeded $150 million. I was in my element, working my butt off but enjoying the challenge.

Then there was the politics. If all politics is local then local politics can be quite the experience. Even when you watch your back, things can get rough. I have the scars to prove it. The occasional negative article or critical editorial is par for the course. It stings when you see it in print, but you get used to it.

As time went on, I developed a good reputation as a solid professional, but at the end of my three-year term year as administrator, there was a shift in political leadership and I was out. Turned out, I was only gone for a year as control shifted back and the re-established majority asked me to leave the government relations position at a water utility where I had landed and return to the county. Despite the politics, I loved the work, so I agreed. This time, the climate was extremely different and the politics became a major intrusion on my professionalism. I found myself in the crossfire of two battles, the target of threats and insinuations, all playing out on the pages of the local newspapers. I even had derogatory posters nailed to the trees along my running route (true story). In the end, it was just some very intense politics and an extremely valuable learning experience that would stick with me for the rest of my career.

Years after leaving the county and then running my own consulting practice, I was fortunate to get a good amount of some very positive press. The flattering coverage continued when I later became a vice president at the community college in the county where I had been the administrator years before. The positive stories and favorable editorials proved to be extremely meaningful and gratifying as I reflected on the tough times when the press and politicians had hung me out to dry on various occasions. To me, this personal comeback and public reaffirmation confirmed the value of one's ability to hang-tough when adversity hits, no matter how hard. In my case, it was my healthy behavior that served as my personal lifeline during these periods of stress and professional challenge. Running, hitting the ab machine, and a diet centered on portion control combined to keep me feeling good, staying focused, and resilient in the face of political pressures.

After a little more than three years at the college, I had an opportunity to join the executive team at one of the area's leading hospital systems. It was an offer I couldn't turn down. Over the years, I had known a number of their executives, but, most significantly, had come to know their board chairman. As a businessperson and political leader in the region, he was familiar with my work and extended me an opportunity to join the team where I've been for the past six years and currently serve as a senior vice president.

Timing is everything. My move into healthcare came at a point of enormous transformation in both the delivery of care and how we measure our nation's health. Contemporary approaches like population health, among other things, place considerable focus on behavior and social influences, as our nation grapples with enormous expenditure for healthcare, yet alarming rates of obesity and chronic disease persist. 50+ men are at the center of this storm.

As an executive with some 40 years in diversified settings, I've come to value leadership. It comes in all forms, emerging under varied circumstances. Men's health, particularly for men over 50, is in desperate need of leadership and new ideas. I will describe in the pages that follow the confluence of factors in this nation, which I believe represent a tipping point for cultural reform that can transform healthy behavior in 50+ men from the exception to the norm. My personal and professional lives have directly benefited from such behavior. I want others to share this experience. I want to lead.

## The Psychology

Is there anything to my experience of finding solace in healthy behavior? It turns out there is. The science suggests that, in general, social support can promote health behavior and alleviate stress. Further, as I described in Chapter 2, there is specific science that points to self-directed behavior as among the strongest and most sustaining pathways to positive behavior change.

Noted psychologist Sheldon Cohen is an award-winning and longstanding scholar who has advanced theories regarding the influence of social relationships on health. His work has established the influence that social environments have on stimulating positive health behavior. In a seminal article, Cohen (Cohen, 2004) describes his theory of stress buffering and, among other things, suggests that social support may not only alleviate the impact of stress but also facilitate healthful behaviors such as exercise, personal hygiene, proper nutrition, and rest.

In my case, the social support was self-directed and more specifically reflective of Self-Determination Theory (SDT). My gravitation to running and eventually a regular gym routine of running, strength training, and stretching, was not the result of a good friend's advice, a therapist's counsel, or my physician's directive. No, my response to stress was intrinsic. It encompassed the three characteristics required by SDT: (1) it was autonomous (I initiated the behavior on my own), (2) I demonstrated competence in my ability to produce the outcomes I sought, and (3) I felt connected and respected by others by choosing this path.

I cite these theories to demonstrate the wider applicability and validity for all men. For me, it was instinctual, not scientific. I got lucky.

## Today

As I look back on the progression of my personal and professional life, I see a parallel with Angela Duckworth's theory of "Grit" (Duckworth, 2016) and her conclusion that grit gets stronger with age. In my early 20s, I had the motivation of a young man who wanted to look good, have fun through sports, and continue an adult version of his youthful behavior. Entering marriage and moving from my late 20s into my 30s is when the reality of life hit like a thunderbolt. A stillborn child, parenthood, divorce, and some very public professional animosity prompted a completely new reason to live healthily. It was a means of survival, a release from the oppression that came with maturity.

When I passed into my 40s, there was more coping and certainly continued work-related pressure, but with single parenthood came an entirely new form of inspiration. The boys were my world, and I needed to be up to the test in all dimensions of life. Following the trials and tribulations of parenthood are the rewards that come with the success of your children and the extreme satisfaction that it brings. As the boys grew to become adults, our relationships grew to new dimensions that began to merge with the aging process. Weddings, job searches, house shopping, and grandchildren become the focal point.

As I moved into my 50s and 60s, the level of grit increased. A supportive wife has taken my dietary practices to a wonderful new level, with attention to detail like never before. Exercise is more frequent, more intense, and more fun. My boys and I will occasionally workout together and are very much engaged in the exchange of diet tips, healthy menus, and health-related practices. This all occurs within the context of an active social calendar. Boys'-night-out dinners, trips to Las Vegas to celebrate birthdays, and NFL talk now highlight my relationship with the boys. It yields a new aspect of social interaction and enjoyment, and continued inspiration to be there for them.

These days, I'm up early and more committed to healthy behavior than I can ever remember. My routine is everything. It's with me day to day, on vacation, and on business trips. I've made it portable. No, I'm not ready to run a marathon, climb Everest, or enter the next triathlon, but I feel good as I approach each day, and what the future holds inspires me.

So, is my passion the product of my experiences? Could I have gotten here without the pain and adversity? I'd guess not. Life doesn't work that way for Everyman. For us, it's a lot of trial and error and rolling with life's punches. What I hope my stories demonstrate is the power of motivation, the strength that emotional and personal factors represent for men, and the benefits one can derive. My experiences may or may not match yours, and yours may certainly be more challenging. What I do hope you see is that healthy behavior is all about achieving the endgame, your life's priorities, and being there for your loved ones. That's what it's been for me. Let me leverage my battle scars and show you how to design your own lifestyle architecture.

## Social Motivation: 10 Strategies for Developing Your Lifestyle Architecture

The men in my research have charted a course for sustained motivation for living a healthy lifestyle. They anchor their path to a strong cognitive alignment between their most valued priorities and their behavior. Day to day, they employ a number of tactics that translate their motivation into actions, tailored to their individual circumstances, but grounded in a common body of inspiration: their lifestyle architecture. They found an added level of confidence in the consistency of this psychological and social approach to health with some of psychology's major theories.

The model is there. Now it's your turn to create your own individual lifestyle architecture. To guide you in your design, I offer 10 strategies gleaned from the stories of the 50+ men I interviewed and my experiences. These stories illustrate the strategies and add a human dimension for deeper meaning. Exercises at the conclusion of each chapter drive home the concepts and will help you jump-start your planning.

The first three strategies are the building blocks for your design. They are a prerequisite for any successful plan, providing an opportunity for you (and hopefully others in your life) to seriously consider your priorities and aspirations, as well as the optimal pathways to achieve your goals. With this foundation, Strategies 4 through 10 offer key design elements, again, emerging from my research and personal experience. In all cases, the strategies are a composite of social factors and behaviors woven together to create the strength you'll need for sustainability.

Here's a look at what's ahead:

1.  **Assess Your Current State**
    All good plans start with a candid and introspective assessment of your present state of social circumstances

and health behavior. Answering the question "Where are you now?" is fundamental to a successful plan.

2.  **Create Your Vision**

    Once you acknowledge your current state, you can consider, "Where do you want to be?" Goal setting is the first step in translating your social vision into concrete, measurable actions that will form sustainable inspiration.

3.  **Build Your Strategy**

    Your implementation strategy, what I characterize in the question: "How are you going to get there?" is where the rubber meets the road. It's your daily, weekly, monthly, and annual action plan, which fuels your inspiration and implements your plan.

4.  **Create Your Personal Lifestyle Network**

    Partnerships and social engagement are a common theme among men who live healthily. This strategy guides you in the development of your own social network.

5.  **Design A Sustainability Plan**

    Contingency planning is common in business and life. It should also be part of your personal health behavior. The healthily-behaving men have a plan. You'll need to consider this for your lifestyle design.

6.  **Leverage Micromotivators**

    While your lifestyle design appropriately starts with consideration of your biggest, or macro, values and priorities, your micromotivators are what serve as the support structure in the practical details of your daily routines. I'll offer several perspectives on identifying microsources of inspiration.

7. **Diversify**

   Just like your financial portfolio, a diversity of social and behavioral tactics adds strength and security to your lifestyle architecture.

8. **Be Optimistic**

   There is a link between optimism and good health. I'll explain the value of optimism and show you how you can learn to be optimistic.

9. **Adjust**

   Life is not a stagnant proposition. Circumstances, values, and behaviors can and sometimes need to change, particularly as you age. Adjusting to new ideas and circumstances is a key factor in your design.

10. **Be A Hero**

    Knowing that we can influence the behavior of others by our actions, whether they are our 50+ brothers or the next generation of men, can be a powerful motivator.

# 4

# Assess Your Current State

IT'S A WIDELY HELD opinion in psychology, particularly in the study of relationships, that men are the gender typically associated with problem-solving and fixing things. We are less concerned with emotional support. Talking through the underlying details of a conflict and other dimensions of the human condition are more commonly associated as the purview of women. Men see solutions as a means to protect their women and loved ones. Their focus on outcomes is how they express their concern. Conversely, women give more weight to processes.

My instinct, as an executive, is to use the power of leverage to achieve goals. I also know that message framing is central to acceptance and adoption of a desired behavior. As you embark on the first of my 10 strategies for designing your lifestyle architecture, answering the question, "Where Are You Now?" on the healthy behavior and social alignment scale, I want to offer a conceptual framework to anchor your thinking. The concept is itself motivating, aligned with the psychosocial insights of my research and consistent with a man's need to fix things.

This predisposition with problem-solving, a man's obsession with protecting that which he values with a quick fix, represents a context to advance the state of men's health. Using a man's inherent need to fix leverages this instinctive mindset on his own behavior. As you've learned from the healthily living men, they align their healthy lifestyle with a mindset of protecting and supporting those for whom they care most. The men I studied expressed that healthy behavior supports a wide range of benefits to the individuals and activities that they value most. If men can close the gaps in their own health behaviors, a multitude of positive outcomes fall into place: a more active social life with their spouse/partner and increasingly robust relationships with their children and grandchildren, as well as professional and other social engagements.

My point is simple. I believe that a man's instinctual interest in problem-solving is translatable to advance his healthy behavior. If alleviating the day-to-day problems that arise in our relationships makes you feel good or satisfy a need in your soul, think of the potential benefits of a healthy lifestyle. It's the ultimate fix!

## The Design Criteria

The men I studied have provided a design template for finding motivation in social factors and transferring that motivation into behavior. I referred to backward reasoning earlier, offering a model that shows how healthy behaving men view their priorities, where they find inspiration, and the tactics they use to carry out their lifestyles. With that model available for reference, your first strategy is to assess your own level of awareness and reconcile your current state with that model.

## Where Are You Now?

When it comes to your most valued priorities, what's your level of awareness? How present are those priorities in your thinking? Are they a source of motivation? Do you exhibit Male Cognitive Behavior Alignment? These and other questions form the heart of my approach to men's health and represent the starting point in the design of your lifestyle architecture. Once you have established a solid understanding, you'll then move to goal setting (i.e., "Where Do You Want to Be?")

in the next chapter, followed by your implementation strategies (i.e., "How Are You Going to Get There?") in Chapter 6. This sequence will help you build the foundation of your lifestyle architecture and from there, you'll move on to reinforcement and additional supportive strategies.

With any planning exercise in business or elsewhere, the process starts with an assessment of your current state, the extent to which you meet the criteria for healthy behavior, how you think about your health, and how much consideration to give to the consequences of your behavior in terms of your life's aspirations. The exercises at the end of the chapter will spur thought and drive home the points you'll need to build your lifestyle architecture. In advance of these exercises, let's walk through some of the thinking behind the process.

The question "Where Are You Now?" has five key dimensions, (1) your current behaviors, (2) your values, (3) your priorities, (4) your motivations, and (5) your tactics. You serve your best interest by answering in the most honest terms. There is no right or wrong answer. It's about identifying your current state as accurately as possible. Remember, you can't fix what you don't perceive as a problem. This is truly a case where honesty IS the best policy.

### Current Health Behaviors

We start with the screening questions that determine whether you currently live a healthy lifestyle. The exercise poses the same five questions used to identify the men I studied. It will enable you to level-set, providing a high-level picture of how you fare on the behavioral scale. If you score a perfect five out of five, congratulations, you are living a healthy lifestyle. The strategies that follow can help you sustain your behavior. If not, the answers will help you begin to focus on the gaps in your architecture.

Among the five questions is one concerning BMI or Body Mass Index, a widely used measure of health. Like many measures, BMI is not without its critics, a point I learned firsthand from my interview with Dr. Geoffrey Williams at the University of Rochester, which you'll read about later.

According to the National Institute of Health, BMI is a useful measure of overweight and obesity. It uses your height and weight to calculate an estimate of body fat. It serves as a good gauge of your risk for diseases that can occur with more body fat. The higher your BMI, the higher your risk for certain diseases such as heart disease, high blood pressure, type 2 diabetes, gallstones, breathing problems, and certain cancers. Although both men and women use the BMI, it does have some limits. It may overestimate body fat in athletes and others who have a muscular build. It may underestimate body fat in older persons and others who have lost muscle.

Readings under 18.5 classify as underweight. A BMI between 18.5 and 24.9 is normal, 25 to 29.9 overweight, and a BMI of 30 or above classify as obese.

CT scans and MRIs can provide a clearer glimpse, but are expensive and involved compared to stepping on a scale. Dual-energy X-ray absorptiometry (DEXA) images are also costly. Researchers have been pushing for using waist circumference, or even wrist circumference, to gauge potentially harmful weight gain and fat depots, but the evidence supporting this measurement and its ability to predict future health problems isn't definitive enough yet. All this considered, BMI remains a directional tool to being one's journey and doesn't preclude you from utilizing these alternative measures as you advance.

## Values and Priorities

The remaining questions, beginning with values and priorities, are the same I posed to the men I surveyed. They make up an inventory of your thoughts on your most valued priorities and the degree to which these values impact your health behavior. Overwhelmingly, the healthily living men showed a high degree of awareness that translated into positive behavior. What are your priorities? How often do you reflect on their importance to you? Have you ever conducted your own inventory and considered the consequences of a poor state of health and your personal aspirations?

This is where the proverbial rubber meets the road. Too often men compartmentalize their priorities and associate them with certain aspects of their lives: earning a living, a roof over their heads, and food on the table. But there's more. If we're going to be there for them: the children, grandchildren, foster children, big brothers, professional colleagues, and the like—you need to consider yourself, drag these priorities into the realm of your own lifestyles, and find the cognitive alignment present in the lifestyle model. Do you have a clear picture of your priorities? Does this image provide motivation? These and other questions will prompt the level of introspection required to tap into the emotional anchors that can form the awareness you need.

## Motivations and Tactics

The final two keys of your personal assessment help you to identify your sources of motivation and any habits, routines, or rituals you employ to sustain your health behaviors. Our social relationships, activities, and plans are how you operationalize your priorities and fuel your continuing cycle of motivation. How robust is your social calendar? Does your social agenda reflect your priorities? What degree of alignment between your valued relationships, if any, is present in your social calendar over the past year? The men I spoke to have a full calendar and thrive on their activities. It gives them purpose and a reason to live healthily.

## MCBA

Beyond the five core dimensions of your assessment, there is another factor that I'd suggest that you consider: Male Cognitive Behavioral

Alignment (MCBA; or—the degree to which you integrate your behavioral and social activities.) Do you work out or eat regularly with a loved one or a friend? I've already introduced a few of the men who do. Throughout the course of the book, you'll see stories reflecting the coupling of healthy behaviors and social goals. Your placement on this scale is another important part of your personal inventory.

## The Design Elements: Recap

If a man's instinct to solve problems is an expression of his concern for the ones he cares about most, then fixing his own behavior, (the most significant impact on his health) can be a home run. When viewed through the prism of motivation, it's all a matter of cognitive alignment among these instincts, the underlying emotions, and the consequences of behavior. You now have your orientation.

With this foundation, you can embark on the process of inventorying your lifestyle and evaluating your results against the template designed by the men. I hope that the logic of the problem-solving argument and the depth of the questions in the exercise will strike the emotional cord that triggers the motivation you seek. However, to increase the chances that you'll consider the seriousness of the proposition, I will supplement this logic-based approach with an emotionally based one, since fear was the most significant motivator among the men I surveyed.

## HEALTHY BEHAVIOR START-UP

| TRADITIONAL APPROACH | SOCIAL MOTIVATION APPROACH |
|---|---|
| Visit your primary care physician | Assess your current state of behaviors against the five-point healthy behavior criteria. |
| Identify a weight-reduction target | Perform an in-depth inventory of your social and emotional priorities in in life; rank those that you value most. |
| Purchase gym membership, equipment | Consider the consequences of your health behaviors, or lack thereof, in the context of your life's aspirations; measure your level of Male Cognitive Behavior Alignment. |
| Hire a trainer | Reflect on your level of social reinforcement. What's the extent of your social activity to build and sustain your social motivation? |
| Purchase workout gear | Create a personal vision for each of your most important relationships |
| Identify a diet plan | Develop a year-round plan of social activity tied to this diet as a means to fortify your level of motivation |
| Check your weight | Continually look for new social motivators and use them to strengthen your motivation platform |

Figure 7: Traditional vs Crack the Code

## Beyond the Logic: Fear as a Motivator

Some men intuitively grasp the behavior-consequence relationship. Just the thought of losing their functionality and independence is enough to prompt good behaviors. Still, many come to this understanding because of unique encounters with fear and their own personal wake-up-call for lifestyle change. Regardless of the pathway, a common destination among the men I questioned is a personal declaration of independence, spurred by an awareness of the behavior-consequence relationship, producing an internalized commitment to healthy behavior.

While loss of personal independence is certainly a major motivational dimension in itself, the survey responses demonstrate that the fears of these men link closely to the loss of their most valued activities in life. The men internalize this connection and view healthy behavior as an insurance policy against the loss. The strength of this connection provides a valuable lesson to men looking for motivation.

## Categories of Fear

The classification of these fears provides further insight into the role that fear plays in stimulating motivation for behavior change (Jarrett, 2008). One perspective that I've noted in my research is a two-dimensional categorization I call "realized and unrealized fears." In either case, the fear is sufficient to produce consideration for behavior change (Jarrett, 2008).

I define realized fears as those stemming from actual or "realized" experiences of the man. Such experiences can range from a disease diagnosis to other serious encounters including accidents, debilitating illness, or the like. Realized fears can equally stem from emotional or social factors, such as a cancer scare that proved to be negative, the death or debilitation of a friend or family member, or even something like the loss of a tennis match that causes an individual to rethink his ability to compete as he ages. Regardless of the origination, the fear comes from an actual experience and is of such significance that it triggers a concern in the man and motivates changed behavior.

Unrealized fears are just that, fears whose origins are based on a less personal, more broadly based, and plausible scenarios (i.e., "If I don't lose weight I may develop diabetes.") Here the perception is that unhealthy behaviors or other social factors left unchecked or unaddressed will increase the likelihood of an event or circumstance that becomes a realized fear and cause for behavior change.

The stories that follow provide examples of realized and unrealized fear among the men I interviewed. Their accounts substantiate the role of these fears in generating behavioral change, and specifically healthy living.

## — Alan's Confrontation With His Fears —

Alan is 63-years old. He is the father of two children, a husband, and a former professional dancer. His is a story of realized fear. Alan toured the country doing ballet, tap, and jazz dancing in national tours including *Peter Pan* and *Disney on Parade* until he decided to stop, as he describes it, "cold turkey" because of a problem he was experiencing with throat reflux.

In about 2000, when Alan was somewhere in his late 40s or early 50s, one day he found himself at his daughter's soccer tournament— using a walker, "I'll never forget it; I went to a soccer tournament with my daughter. I had to go with a walker. I had pulled my back out really bad."

According to his doctors, when Alan stopped dancing, it caused his muscles to shrink and become weak. This triggered a severe back problem that required him to use a walker to get around. That day at the soccer tournament turned out to be a significant moment in Alan's life. It triggered an enormous sense of fear, both the fear of losing his independence and the fear that his physical limitations would infringe on his ability to enjoy a fulfilling and active life with his wife and children. As he stood there with his walker, barely 50 years old, watching his daughter run up and down the field and the other parents cheering on their children, Alan faced his fears head-on. "That was the first thing that motivated me," he said.

For a man who had been in such great shape for so many years, the prospect of depending on the walker for his mobility was frightening. That day at the soccer tournament became Alan's transformational moment, his declaration of independence. The awareness that came upon him provided the motivation to embark on a new set of behaviors to address his physical needs, as well as his desire to be there for his growing children. Fortunately, for Alan, he could manage his physical condition. His dependence on the walker ended with the full restoration of his ability to walk normally.

After reading a book recommended by one of the "soccer dads" who appeared to be in great shape, Alan began to exercise regularly and watch his diet, which included eliminating dairy. "That's how it all started," he told me. He inspired his wife and daughter to pursue their own healthy practices, making healthy behavior a family affair. However, Alan's story doesn't end there.

About 10 years later, Alan found himself in another fearful situation. Severe chest pains prompted a 911 call and an ambulance trip to the hospital. Alan thought he was having a heart attack. Adding to his fear was the fact that his father had suffered a heart attack when Alan was younger. He thought his fate was to do the same. It turned out to be a throat reflux condition and not a heart problem. Nevertheless, the scare was enough to heighten Alan's already strong commitment to healthy behavior. He became even more diligent about his diet, in part to fight the reflux but also to support his overall health. He has an exercise program that he developed that includes movements of ballet, yoga, and Pilates. He is also dairy and gluten free and maintains a low acid diet.

Most importantly, he has fully internalized his behaviors, enjoys his healthy lifestyle, and cannot imagine living any differently. He will tell you that he has never felt better. While retired from the professional stage, Alan is active in community theater and serves as host and master of ceremony at local civic events.

Alan is fortunate. His brush with incapacitation was not permanent, and his diagnosis of the reflux condition relieved his fear of having a cardiac condition like the one his father had. Still, he came face to face with his fear and leveraged it as motivation to embark on a healthy lifestyle. While the genesis of Alan's motivations appears external, it is clear he has internalized them. He enjoys his healthy lifestyle, and the benefits they provide re-fuel his passion for health. His willingness to extend his practices to include yoga, and his ability to maintain the behaviors for well over a decade now, confirms the strength of his motivation.

Alan's story demonstrates the power of fear as a motivator for healthy behavior and supports the opinions of men in the survey. While his story illustrates an actual confrontation with potentially debilitating events, the good news is that there is no need for you to go through the same process to leverage fear as a source of inspiration. Serious reflection on the behavior-consequence relationship in your own life has the potential to serve the purpose just fine. Let's look at an example of such unrealized fear.

## — Bob's Desire for Functional Fitness —

"I don't want to wake up knowing I'm going to have trouble walking during the day," said Bob in our interview. Bob is a 65-year-old fundraiser who works with non-profit organizations and whose two grandchildren live with him and his wife. An army veteran, his concern over what his life would be like without good health epitomizes the unrealized fear model. While he has never had any serious encounters with his health, he is very much aware of the value of good health in his life.

Bob and his wife live in a three-level home, where everyone is constantly going up and down the steps. He loves to golf and has a habit of walking the course during the nine holes he regularly plays:

> "Functional fitness" is the new buzzword I've seen on line. It means you want to be fit enough to get through the daily functions of life, carrying groceries from the car, if you have kids, interacting with the kids or, in our case, grandchildren.

After discharge from the Army as a young man, Bob realized that he was straying from the fitness regimen he had developed while in the service and didn't like how he felt. From that point forward, Bob adopted a healthy lifestyle, which today includes distance swimming and regular trips to the local YMCA. "When I go to the gym I feel like I'm making a deposit for my future—my future health and fitness."

Whether it's playing basketball with his 12-year-old granddaughter or tending to the backyard with his wife, Bob fears the plight of others his age who are much less engaged in healthy behaviors and visibly pay the price with reduced opportunities to undertake what he enjoys regularly. Yes, while the basis of Bob's fears is a strong aversion to the lifestyle limitations he sees in others his age, the strength of his commitment is equal to what we saw in Alan, demonstrating the power of fear, no matter what pathway it takes up the mountain of motivation.

## Action Planning for Designing Your Own Lifestyle Architecture

Your health is personal; in fact, it is as personal as it gets. This point should ring loudly now that you've diligently read my findings: the wisdom shared by stories of our 50+ men who live healthily and the strategies I've presented to guide you in designing your own lifestyle architecture, built on a foundation of a strong cognitive alignment between your values and behavior. Now, I want to give you the tools to extend this guidance directly into your own life, so that you can enjoy the social and physical benefits of healthy living.

The exercises that follow put my 10 strategies into action for you and Everyman. They will enable you to customize your social approach and tailor the strategies that fit your life. They're intention is to prompt you to look both inward at your most intimate feelings and values, as well as outward at your social relationships and the resources that you can bring to bear on the design of your new lifestyle architecture. While intentionally serious, the exercises can also prove to be fun and something you can engage in with others in your life. If you anchor your motivation in your relationship with others, it may help to bring them into the process. Think in terms of creating your own personal design team.

Following this chapter, I start with the three strategies that form the foundation of your lifestyle design and ask you to consider, "Where are you now?", "Where do you want to be?", and "How are you going to get there?" Exercise 1 poses some of the same questions we gave our men. See how you fare. The tables that follow in the subsequent exercises are a visual guide to organize your thoughts. Feel free to use your own means of recording your answers. The key is to keep a log of your responses, as they will come in handy in the later chapters. Strategies 4 through,10 build on this foundation by adding supporting elements and techniques I gleaned from the men, as well as from my own experiences. Think of them as additional infrastructure in the architecture that will help you sustain your behavior and continually revisit your plans as circumstances change.

As a leader in men's health, my goal is to help you maximize the quality of your life. In the case of the 50+ men, I believe that these social strategies and a focus on motivation represent a new and exciting way to approach healthy behavior. I encourage you to make the most of these tools. Go for it!

## Conclusion

I am a big believer in getting off to a good start and tackling the most challenging issues up front. In this context, it means you honestly assess the current state of your behavior, priorities, and awareness of the consequences associated with your lifestyle. Regardless of whether you ultimately find your motivation for a healthy lifestyle by its appeal to your problem-solving instincts, the logic of the behavioral-consequences argument, or fear is immaterial. You just need to find it and that process starts with your personal inventory.

Alan and Bob showed us how they turned their fears into a lifestyle of commitment to health. Alan's brush with potentially debilitating medical problems spurred his path, while Bob's unrealized fear triggered his lifestyle changes, should he not maintain his commitment grounds his healthy behavior. Through different routes, each man found his way to positive behavior. Now they are feeling great and enjoying the benefits. The experiences of Alan and Bob highlight the power of emotion. Their stories demonstrate how such emotions operationalize into everyday living.

I encourage you to complete the exercises that follow. You can do them in short order but, importantly, they will spur your thinking and personal reflection. By design, this exercise is the most extensive as it is the most foundational—all the next steps in designing your lifestyle architecture, built upon the feelings and perceptions produced here. Your plan is about to unfold.

# Chapter 4 Exercises

Chapter 4 is about assessing where you are now on two dimensions: your health behaviors and consciousness of your social priorities. As a simple step on the pathway to your personalized plan for social motivation, take a shot at the two exercises below. Be honest and thoughtful. An accurate appraisal of your current state is the foundation for the strategies that follow.

## Step 1: Complete the Health Behavior Questionnaire

Do you lead a healthy lifestyle? I used the following five questions to identify healthily living men for our studies. Start your personal assessment by completing the questionnaire. Circle yes or no next to each question. To calculate your BMI (body mass index) just do a quick internet search for a BMI calculator. A link will pop up fast and then just enter your height and weight and the calculator will give you your BMI. I included one site to make it extra easy.

| HEALTHY BEHAVIORS | | |
|---|---|---|
| I eat fruits and vegetables regularly | YES | NO |
| I exercise for at least 20 minutes a day, three or more days a week | YES | NO |
| I do not smoke | YES | NO |
| I wear a seatbelt when I am in the car | YES | NO |
| I have a healthy BMI | YES | NO |
| *How to calculate a healthy BMI (18.5 - 24.9)<br>  ○  What is your height and weight?<br>  ○  _____ Feet _____ Inches _____ Pounds<br>Input your height and weight into this BMI calculator online<br>http://www.smartbmicalculator.com | | |

Figure 8: Personal Assessment Questionnaire and BMI Index

The healthy men scored five out of five. How did you score? If you answered YES to all five, congratulations, you live a healthy lifestyle. The strategies that follow can help you sustain that behavior. If not, the items where you answered NO represent the gaps you'll need to close to achieve a healthy lifestyle, and, as I learned from the healthy men, looking upstream at social motivators is a great place to start.

## Disclaimer: Smoking & Seat Belt Use

Two of the questions, smoking and seat belt use, represent behaviors that in some ways reside outside the immediate realm of this book. My survey, illustrations, and stories are exclusive to diet, exercise, and physical activity. My focus is largely on social strategies that assist men with motivation for diet and exercise and the resulting impact on BMI. There are no references to smoking and seat belt use.

That said, I would argue that by strengthening a man's social motivations, the cognitive alignment between his values and his behavior, and by providing guiding tactics that could be applied to one's efforts to quit smoking or adopt seat belt use, that these two factors are indeed addressed, albeit indirectly. Social motivators can be equally applicable to smoking and seat belt use as they are behaviors that can significantly increase a man's ability (or reduce the potential of his inability) to fulfill his aspirations with regard to his most valued priority. With this in mind, let's move to Step 2.

## Step 2: Assessing Your Social Motivators

Consider the following questions as a means to assess your priorities, motivations, and strategies. There are no right or wrong answers. I designed these questions to stimulate your thinking, produce a comprehensive assessment of the alignment of your values and behaviors, and give you a comparison against the healthy men.

- What are your priorities in life?

- How conscious are you of your most valued relationships?

- How frequently do you consider these relationships?

- How would you rank your priorities?

- Do they serve as a source of motivation? Are they social or from another source?

- What are your strongest sources of motivation?

- How reinforcing of these relationships is your social calendar?

- What are your greatest fears when it comes to the state of your health?

- Do you use any habits, routines, or rituals to maintain a healthy lifestyle?

## Summary

I hope that these questions have you thinking. It all begins with awareness. From your completion of Step 1, you now know if you're leading a healthy lifestyle. If yes, what can you do to ensure that you sustain these practices? If not, what behaviors do you need to adopt?

In Step 2, consider what you've learned about yourself, your values, and your priorities from the social questions. Do you have some thoughts on how you can strengthen the alignment between your values and your behavior? Do you have a better sense of the specific factors that prompt an emotional response and, consequently, a stronger potential to produce motivation for healthy living? You now have a full picture of your current state, strengths, and gaps in your level of social motivators. With this in hand, you can now build your goals, Strategy #2. Press on.

# 5

## Create Your Vision

THE NEXT PLANK OF your behavior platform concerns goal setting. Any plan, especially one designed to produce motivation for healthy behavior, needs a clear statement of where you want to be in life: your aspirations, ambitions, and dreams. It's basic to any organized effort to ensure your success. As in any strategy, you need quantifiable and measurable goals, described in sufficient detail so that there is no misunderstanding as to what they mean and whether they've been accomplished, in part or in whole. Many people refer to these as SMART goal: specific, measurable, attainable, relevant, and time-bound.

To maximize your opportunities to stimulate motivation, it helps to periodically give yourself a report card on your goals and be able to assess the underlying factors behind your self-determined grades. You can grade yourself on a curve and adjust as appropriate. Regardless, the absence of any benchmarks or defined goals is a recipe for a succession of missed attempts and frustrations at reaching your life's goals and dreams. Therefore, you need a mechanism, a scorecard, to track your performance.

In this chapter, I'll show you how to find your own personalized goals and build your scorecard. Now, the goals I'm referring to don't represent pounds to be shed, sit-ups to crunch, or miles to run. That comes later. No, the goals I'm talking about are those high-level, endgame measures that reflect the very personal and social outcomes that fuel YOUR motivation, which, in turn, produces the lifestyle behaviors you want to maintain.

If the central premise to creating motivation is the ability to link behavior with the attainment of personal and social values, you need to have a deep and meaningful understanding of those values. While this may seem like an obvious connection, it's not. Too many of us engage so deeply in our daily lives we overlook that which is right in front of us. A deep and meaningful understanding means that you have really considered what's important in your life. It means that you have prioritized these factors and treat them with the respect and care that they deserve. Do you ever find yourself immersed in the most trivial nonsense while ignoring things that are more important? Anything worthwhile deserves the appropriate attention.

### Lessons from the Men: The Link is Strong, The Priorities Are Clear, and The Motivation is Consistent

The men I surveyed were very clear about the link between priorities and motivation, as well as the sources of their motivations and the benefits of their lifestyles.

The link is strong. As I mentioned in Chapter 3, 76% said that their priorities play a major role in providing motivation to maintain a healthy lifestyle and 74% think about their priorities quite often.

Their motivations are consistent. We saw that fear and fear-related outcomes are the major source of motivation, but the drill down shows that the fears closely align with the factors at risk, which brings us back to the life priorities. This further aligns with the second tier of top motivating factors, which concerns a man's relationship with his spouse or significant other at 56%. Overall, the men's priorities represent their top motivating factor, with 66% of the men surveyed rating it as their number one motivating factor.

The benefits are clear. The men's perceived benefits of behavior run parallel to these priorities and motivations. The highest ranked benefit of a healthy lifestyle, the absence of debilitating illness, comes in at 96% and maintaining independence at 95%. These align logically with the fear as a top motivator and spouse or significant other as a top priority.

When viewed in the strategic context of goal setting, the findings tell a story. Men who engage in healthy behaviors have values anchored in their life's priorities. These values and their perceived benefits of attaining and sustaining their value-laden activities is the fuel that powers their motivation, which enables and sustains their positive behaviors. For men seeking to adopt such an approach and ultimately internalize the associated behaviors, goal setting and the quality and thoughtfulness that go into the selection of your goals is crucial.

## Thinking About Your Goals

We all think about how we would like our future to play out. As human beings, we need love, comfort, acknowledgement for our actions, and fulfillment in any number of ways. Behavioral scientists are clear on this score. It is basic psychology. The degree to which you meet your needs influences your happiness and ultimately your ability to produce the motivation that supports desired behavior. This relationship is at the core of intrinsic motivation.

By studying the attributes of healthy men, I reached two conclusions. The first is that the starting point for building the connection between psychological needs and motivation is a deep and meaningful understanding of a man's priorities and values. Second, is that motivation is a very personal issue. I interviewed men motivated by experiences that range from shooting hoops with their granddaughters, to travel with their wives, to business pursuits. Their strategies for healthy living include swimming the equivalent of the English Channel in multiple trips to the pool at the local YMCA—to chopping wood—to eating salmon. They maintain a very conscious awareness that these experiences make them feel good, which in turn produces the motivation to sustain the behavior. Bottom line, they enjoy and benefit from the behavior.

## Shaping Your Goals

Now is the time to start shaping your goals. This is your first of many defining moments. It's your opportunity to take yourself and your loved ones to another level. By personalizing and applying my findings, you can begin the process of developing your own lifestyle architecture. This is indeed a process, as these priorities will refine along the way and even change dramatically with time and experience.

For starters, take some time to reflect and really think about yourself, your goals, and your priorities. Jot down what comes to mind, as if you were here sitting with me discussing your life's aspirations. What would you list as being significant enough to motivate you to make changes in your life? Use the following questions to stimulate your thinking.

- Do you want to be there for your family in the next five, 10, 15, or 20 years??

- Do you have any fears?

- Do you have a spouse, partner, or loved one with whom you love to spend time?

- What activities give you the most satisfaction in life?

- Do you like to travel?

- Are there activities, challenges, or other things that you've always wanted to do but have not yet accomplished?

- Do you have hobbies?

- Are there milestone events in your life that you're looking forward to (i.e., graduations, weddings, trips retirement, grandchildren)?

- Do you maintain an interest in professional accomplishments?

How do your priorities compare with the men in our survey? My hope is that these questions will enable you to go deep inside and pull out those needs and desires that allow you to understand yourself and discover what's meaningful to you.

Additionally, remember, goal setting need not be a solo act. Engage those you love, trust, or rely on, and they can serve as teammates in your crusade. Consult your spouses, children, physicians, and friends, particularly if they'll play some role in the execution of the goal related activities. Tell the people you are close to that you are entering upon this journey, and you will expand your opportunities for growth while inviting limitless possibilities for you to become the healthiest version of yourself ever!

## Organizing Your Goals

Once you devote yourself to the effort of really understanding what makes you tick, you can begin to organize and prioritize your goals. To guide you in this process, I have provided you with a structured approach that will further stimulate your thinking and allow you to tailor your ambitions to your individual circumstances. I've identified six goal categories that are generic in nature, but are likely to capture your unique aspirations. The categories include personal, spouse/partner, children, grandchildren, social, and professional.

This is by no means an exhaustive list, and you can expand the organization of the categories. If this list does not include your interests, no problem, you can create additional classifications or place your specific ideas in any category you wish. The key is to organize your thoughts and record them. My goal is to provide you with a simple illustration, drawn from the survey findings that will provoke your thought. To maximize the value of this process, record your goals or even potential goals. As you move through the process you may find that there lies an athlete, educator, artist, or businessperson within you that you didn't know existed!

Below is a brief description of each category, along with some examples. They will provide the perspective you need to identify and adopt your own goals in the exercise that follows this chapter. Chapter 6 will then build on this start by taking you through the process of determining how best to implement these goals, and I'll offer an alternative, more refined view, focused on tactics. For now, examine the following categories of goals and begin to consider how they match up with your life and what specifically you would like to accomplish for each.

## Personal Goals

Since goal setting is a very personal expression, it is appropriate that I start here. I consider this a wide-ranging category that can include goals centered on: longevity and maintaining independence, education (i.e., pursuing a degree, taking a class at the local high school, piano lessons, or training of any form), personal development (i.e., writing a book, painting, yoga, acting in local theater), financial security, or hobbies.

## Spouse/Partner Goals

Time spent with a spouse or partner ranked number one among the surveyed men, so I expect that it is highly likely that you will have goals in this category. Travel, social activities, and your sex life are all appropriate targets for this area.

## Children

Time and activities with children is also a highly ranked motivator among the surveyed men and likely to be among your personal goals. We include stepchildren as well as Big Brothers and other volunteer-based programs in this net, either in addition to, or as a substitute for, your own children and a great extension of parenting.

## Grandchildren

Similar to children and particularly as men age, grandchildren are sure to generate a wide range of goals. Writing down these goals is important.

## Professional

There are many dimensions of today's economy that translate into goals for 50+ men. Ambitions centered here include extended careers, second or third careers, part-time opportunities, volunteer-positions, and work-at-home alternatives. Financial need, or simply the desire to remain active in the workforce, often drives professional goals. While not a highly-rated motivator compared to the more personal factors, professional goals remain an important driver for some men.

## Social

We value our social relationships: other couples, friends from work, gym buddies, travel mates, or the sporting event crew. Here, I'll also place non-professional volunteer work, civic engagement, and faith-based activities. As the findings showed, partnerships are important to men. You're probably going to have something to include here.

## Our Men and Their Goals

### — Bob —

Let's go back to Bob, our fundraiser. He and his wife live an active lifestyle, and they have very definitive ideas about things they want to achieve in life. They have goals and strategies that they employ to implement these goals. Most importantly, Bob ties his ability to achieve his goals to his behavior, which in turn produces more motivation to maintain the behavior. The result is a positive cycle of psychological rewards, recycled into more motivation. It all starts with Bob's very specific ideas about where he wants to be at age 65 and the years ahead. He has goals in three of our categories: grandchildren, travel, and professional. Here is what I mean.

As we learned, Bob's two granddaughters, ages eight and 11, the daughters of their son and daughter respectively, live with Bob and his wife. He has very specific goals when it comes to them. Among them is his desire to engage in recreational activities and be a part of their lives:

> When my granddaughter says, "Pop-Pop, let's go down to the Y and shoot some baskets." I can't say my knees hurt or my back hurts. I just say, "Let's go!" That energizes me. My eight-year-old granddaughter is on the swim team at the Y. She's terrific. She's a natural. I watch her practices a couple times a week. It's inspiring to me. How great is this?

Another major priority for Bob and his wife is travel. Bob met his wife in Kentucky, when he was attending the University of Kentucky. She still has family there, so it's a frequent destination for family vacations. For a while, they enjoyed time in Florida where they owned a time-share in Key West, and when Bob was still in the Army, they toured Germany together. Both of Bob's children are finishing their degrees. When they finish, he and his wife expect that they'll have more time for themselves and are already contemplating their travel ideas:

> We like horseback riding. We like canoeing. We like kayaking. We got into snorkeling when we were traveling down the Keys. So, we're saying, "Wow, let's think about doing that again down the road. There's a lot we have planned in the future. My Dad was a pilot in World War II, so one of my goals is to tour airbases in Europe where my Dad served."

Professionally, Bob's goals focus on balancing his continuing desire to earn a living for his family with his interest in giving back to the community. "I've designed my professional life around a quote from Winston Churchill: You make a living by what you earn, you make a life by what you give."

Today, Bob balances his professional time between his leadership of a local Toastmasters organization and the fundraising services he offers, but he guides his pursuits by a clear set of priorities. "I'm still earning a living for my family, but it's of equal priority, if not lower priority, with my other interests."

## — Carmen —

Carmen is 65 and retired from a career in construction. He hasn't had a drink for 30 years and stays away from sweets. He enjoys the benefits of his wellness regimen, which allows him, and his wife to travel together, and provides him the ability to fish with his son and spend time with his three-year-old granddaughter. Personal factors, aspirations for travel with his wife, and spending time with his children and granddaughter are the major goals in his life.

Like many of the men I surveyed, Carmen's very personal goal is to live a long life and maintain his health, so he can enjoy his family:

> Me being healthy makes it so that I'm going to be around for a while. That's what my goal is, to be around for as long as I can be around. As long as I have my grandkids and my wife—we like to travel—as long as I can do that, I want to stay healthy, so I can do it.

Carmen's face lights up when asked about his wife. His relationship with her another major goal, "I have a great relationship with my wife. She's the one who keeps me going. She keeps me on the right path."

A thyroid problem caused Carmen to focus on his health. Today, he hits the high school track several times a week, sometimes twice a day, with his buddy and later with his wife. He likes the way it makes him feel, he likes the way his clothes fit and, most importantly, his ability to keep up with kids increases, another big goal for him.

> I go (to workouts) because I have to be in shape to do that kind of stuff. My son and I, we go out on the rocks. When you are fishing off the rocks, the jetty, you have to be in shape to fish out on those rocks. Yeah, I try to keep up with him. I keep up with him. I like to do whatever they [his children] do. I want to keep myself where I can do the things they do, so I can hang with them.

Carmen sees his children frequently and typically goes out to dinner with them one night per week. According to him, they are all "health nuts" and keep after him about his diet and exercise. Adding to the family-founded inspiration are his grandchildren.

> I get out there and I play ball with my grandkids when they come over and we bar-b-que during the summer. We'll play kickball out in the yard they've got me running the bases and whispering to me, "Hey, Poppy, you run fast for an old guy." The next day I'm hurting but I get it done. It makes me feel great.

Carmen knows where he wants to be for the foreseeable future. Achieving his goals provides him extreme satisfaction and meets his psychological needs. As a result, he has a constant source of motivation to sustain his wellness program.

Bob and Carmen are in a positive cycle of value-driven motivation and beneficial behavior. They have a clear sense of the factors that meet their needs and use the attainment of those goals to deliver the motivation that maintains the cycle. As you can see in these examples, Bob and Carmen have built an awareness in their minds, an awareness that links their most precious and valued factors in life and ties them to behaviors that support their health. This positive cycle is healthy for them and, by extension, their families, and friends. It starts with a deep and personal look inward to examine and identify what's most important to you. With clarity about where you want to be, you can build your own personalized portfolio of goals that will get you on the road to enjoying yourself, just like Bob and Carmen.

## Chapter 5 Exercises

Chapter 5 is about translating your social priorities into concrete goals, which form the foundation of your lifestyle architecture. These goals are high-level statements of your aspirations that you achieve through a series of more specific tactics and strategies covered in the next chapter. For now, the simple step is to answer the question, "Where do I want to be?" in terms of advancing the priorities you've identified as your social motivators.

In this chapter, I've provided you with goal categories and some examples to spur your thinking. Below are some fully stated sample goals, which further drive home the exercise. See if any apply to your life.

When creating your own goals, start small: Try to come up with one or two in each of the categories. You can certainly add more categories and have more goals in each category, but starting slowly and building your portfolio is a good way to begin.

Consult your loved ones and anyone you think can help. Have fun! Remember, you want to establish goals that will provide you with the strongest motivation to live healthily and generate sustained inspiration. Just as you saw in the stories of Bob and Carmen, the goals represent accomplishments that will give your life added purpose, meaning, and satisfaction, and, by doing so, provide the energy and discipline to live healthily.

You're two-thirds of the way to completing the foundation of your lifestyle architecture!

## Sample Social Goals

### Personal Goals

I want to be financially secure in my retirement.

I want to learn how to play the piano.

I want to run a 5K race.

### Spouse/Partner Goals

I want to travel more with my wife.

I want to take my wife dancing every week.

I want to spend more quality time with my wife.

### Children & Related Activities

I want to stay as engaged as I can in my children's lives.

I want to become more engaged in the lives of my niece/nephew.

I want to join the Big Brother or Big Sister Program.

### Grandchildren

I want to see my grandson/daughter graduate from college.

I want to be able to take walks, swim, and enjoy activities with my grandchildren.

I want to dance with my granddaughter at her wedding.

### Professional

I want to work part or full-time.

I want to mentor junior colleagues.

I want to teach.

### Social

I want to maintain and expand my relationships with my social circle of friends.

I want to volunteer in my community.

I want to attend all the games of my favorite professional sports team.

# 6

## Build Your Strategy

RHYTHM. HEALTHY LIFESTYLES HAVE a rhythm and a cadence. The routines, rituals, and habits that translate value-driven goals into day-to-day practices produce this rhythm and form the pathway to achieve your goals. They are the vehicle that gets you to your destination. The practices can be socially oriented activities that sustain your motivation and reinforce the connection between values and behavior or the behavior itself: diet, exercise, or hobbies. Ideally, it's both. I've found this to be true in the men I've interviewed

Either way, the rhythm is good. It's self-policing. Once you get into your rhythm, you don't want to miss a beat. It doesn't feel right. Socially, you don't want to miss your weekly dinner with the kids, that morning walk in the park with your wife, the family vacation, or perhaps even the annual business convention. With behaviors, your workout schedule, dietary practices, and hobbies become second nature. A disruption in the rhythm of these activities is discomforting. You have come to enjoy these practices. They feel good and strengthen the tie back to your values. The elements of your rhythm are bite-sized actions that maintain your focus, and can actually take your life to a completely new level!

Building rhythm also serves to add structure and the level of personal accountability you want. The social and behavioral objectives used to accomplish broader goals satisfy your need to have discrete and measurable actions (i.e., the SMART goals) to evaluate performance and amend your strategies. Again, all good stuff.

## Habits, Rituals, and Routines Are Common Among Healthy Men

My survey findings confirm the importance of rhythm and the inclusion of both social and behavioral factors in ways men seek to achieve their goals. As I ran down in Chapter 2, 95% of the men have specific habits and rituals and 83% of them find them extremely or very important. Drilling deeper, the research showed that the highest rated routines included hobbies, dining, and engaging in activities with a spouse, family member, or a friend. Meal planning and maintaining a regular schedule for exercise, the avoidance of certain food groups, and portion control were among the top-rated dietary habits.

The pattern is clear. Compile an inventory of social and behavioral activities that support your life priorities and goals, and then work it. Just like a major-league pitcher or any athlete who is having a good outing, you want to get into a groove and establish a rhythm. Intermingling your social and behavioral tactics will strengthen the fabric of your lifestyle, providing you with tremendous benefits. They are the keys to your success and sustainability.

The actions that you select to accomplish your goals are extremely important. It's where the rubber meets the road in your efforts to find motivation for healthy living. To show you exactly how this works, here are two case studies. The first is mine: some examples of how I've created a rhythm on both the social and behavioral sides of my life and how they keep me locked-in on my healthy lifestyle. The second is a story from one of the men I interviewed. Together, they will provide a context and provide you with an example of the detailed strategies you'll need to build your own goal-accomplishing rhythm.

### My Rhythm

I love the rhythm of my lifestyle. I couldn't live without it. It has grown to become a source of pride and satisfaction. It gives me comfort that

I have an organized approach to what's most important in my life. It feels good.

My rhythm includes a morning exercise routine, TGIF night dinners with my wife, and, when I can get them, my adult children, as well as annual trip to Florida with my son for baseball's spring training. They are both social and behavioral. Each example ties to one of my priorities: being there for my family, a solid marriage, and close relationships with my children. The specificity of the actions enables me to easily determine if I've accomplished what I intended. Periodically, I can assess whether these activities contribute to my larger goals. This, in turn, prompts me to consider other activities that might further enhance the attainment of those goals. Most importantly, the actions serve as a year-long ongoing wellspring of inspiration, rewards, and continual motivation.

## Behavioral Activities That Help You Reach Your Goal

Here is just one example of what I mean from the behavioral side. I love my morning routine. It's my personal time to reflect on the day ahead and get my exercise. It makes me feel great and gets me ready for what lies ahead every day. During the week, I typically awake at 4 a.m., enjoy a cup of coffee, and shave. While I'm shaving, I'll contemplate the day ahead, what I need to accomplish, and what's outstanding, or particularly challenging. I'll quickly check my overnight email and perhaps add some items to my daily to-do list (another habit that keeps my life in order).

As you might guess, I'm the only one up at this hour. The stillness of the house is peaceful and provides me with a clarity of thought that helps me prepare for the day ahead.

By about 10 minutes to five, I'm on my way to the gym, which is only five minutes away (an important factor). My rhythm stems from a schedule of weight training on Monday, Wednesday, and Friday and cardio workouts on Tuesday, Thursday, and Saturday. I particularly like the cardio days for the good sweat. While running, I'll usually think about the day ahead and use the challenges of the upcoming day to power my run on the treadmill. By 6:00 a.m., I'm on my drive home, stopping to pick up some oatmeal, which I eat while I'm reading my three newspapers (two local and the *Wall Street Journal*). After a shower, it's off to the office. My day is officially underway.

As you can see, there's nothing terribly glamorous here. That's the point of rituals, and what I heard from the men I interviewed reinforced it. While we all have the "big ticket" milestone activities (i.e., the trips to Europe I took with family in 2000 and 2013) that motivate us to maintain our health, but in large measure I find that it's those small day-to-day actions that have the most impact on sustaining behavior and providing inspiration and accomplishment. In my case, six days a week, I have an opportunity to check off a box on my list of personal objectives. Being able to check that box, even mentally, is one small way that I contribute to the larger goal and physically feeling good in the process. You get it.

Do I sometimes miss my morning routine? Absolutely, if I'm not in bed by 9:30 p.m. (preferably nine o'clock) then 4 a.m. doesn't work. So, a late meeting or other commitment can get me out of rhythm and feeling just a little "off" that day. Nevertheless, having institutionalized the practice, my body wants to get back in rhythm the next day, which I'm typically able to do. As much as humanly possible, the morning routine carries on during vacations and business trips. I may waive the 4 a.m. wake-up call for a later hour, but I generally maintain the basic exercise and diet regimen when I'm on the road.

One last caveat: Most recently, my younger son has moved closer and adopted the early morning workout routine at my gym. So now, this dad's in heaven because he gets to see his son almost every day (and daughter-in-law on the weekends). While it's just a short hug and brief conversation (we're both serious about our workouts) it means the world to me and is the ultimate blend of social and behavioral activity. I am blessed.

## A Pyramid of Social Activities

On the social side of my life, I maintain a portfolio of activities that provides a continual source of activity on the horizon and installments toward my larger goals. I think of them as a hierarchical pyramid with four levels. At the base of the triangle, Level One, are the routine social events that comprise the majority of the portfolio. They are the foundation of my social pyramid. More frequent and regimented, they confront the fact that much of life is routine.

In my experience, the ability to breathe excitement and interest into the routine fuels my motivation. I have come to thrive on the routine and find inspiration is the smallest of upcoming plans. Whether it's dinner with my wife on Friday night, seeing my new grandson, a ball game, summer weekends at our beach house, or even an important business event, these are the most basic activities that support the larger goals. They are the daily, weekly, and monthly events that give me the drive and determination to stay active and, ultimately, healthy.

Level Two contains the more significant or "special" installments. Here I include vacations with my wife, upcoming visits from out-of-town family, an occasional lecture, or even household projects. I think of them as a product of what I call "social entrepreneurialism," proactively looking for opportunities to do cool things with my spouse, family, or friends. I typically mine the travel and education sections of the papers and online sources to find ideas.

Level Three is what I label "bonding" experiences. These are unique, often intergenerational events with family, creating bonds that live on for years. We share the stories and traditions at family gatherings and other occasions with fondness and appreciation. They produce a closeness that strikes a bullseye on the target of personal values. In my lifetime, three examples best highlight this category: two family trips to Europe and an annual spring training trip to Florida.

In 2000, I took my dad and two sons to Italy and Croatia for a two-week trip. I was single at the time, and my older son was about to start college. I saw this as an important juncture and a reason to do something special that would be fun and simultaneously create some lifetime memories. Taking the kids to Croatia enabled them to visit their homeland, as our family is Croatian. They were able create some bonds with their grandfather, who spoke the language and still had a cousin in the City of Split. To make a long story short, we had a great time on our "guys' getaway." While the war in the former Yugoslavia was long over, remnants of the conflict remained, and the best hotel I could find still reflected wartime conditions, which were Spartan at best. Today, we laugh about these conditions and talk about how much fun we had swimming in the Adriatic Sea and soaking up our ancestral heritage. It brought us together and provided us with a lifetime of memories.

Fast forward to 2013: I am now married again, as is my oldest son. My dad is about to turn 87, and we decide to celebrate his 87th birthday in Croatia. This time we brought the women: my wife, daughter-in-law, and my dad's longtime significant other. Again, this was a significant bonding experience. And, this time, the hotel was magnificent! The highlight was the birthday party, which my son and daughter-in-law had arranged at a winery outside Split. Between the foods, the wine, and the Jeep ride through the woods (yes, with my 87-year old father and his significant other in a Jeep with us, traversing the countryside), we will never forget this wonderful experience.

My final bonding example is one built around the goal of building traditions. In this case, spring training. For the past five years, and hopefully more in the future, my oldest son and I (we are Phillies fans, and his brother—for reasons I don't quite understand—is a Rangers fan) venture down to Florida for a long weekend of baseball and father and son bonding. Spring training baseball, the Florida sun in March, the pool, great meals, and a little March Madness at the hotel bar—it doesn't get any better. If you haven't tried it, you don't know what you're missing. To say the least, just like Croatia, the excursions and our experiences have given us a wealth of material that has brought my son and me closer.

In the fourth and final level, I place life's milestone events: weddings, births, graduations, and milestone birthdays. If these events don't get you pumped up, I don't know what will. I have been fortunate to have two phenomenal weddings between the boys and a host of graduations. As I write this book, we are in the process of planning my dad's 90th birthday. Talk about milestone events! Whether it's your immediate family, a Big Brother event, or even a close friend, milestone events are cause for celebration and the source of inspiration for the healthy behavior that will get you there.

## PYRAMID OF SOCIAL ACTIVITIES

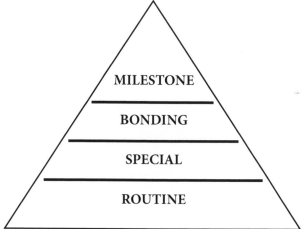

Figure 9: Pyramid of Social Activities

This is a bit of personal experience to give you one man's approach to building rhythm for healthy living through a combination of behavioral and social endeavors. Let's now look at another perspective from one of the men in my study.

## — Health is Wealth —

Vijay is an electrical engineer in his 60s. He has been married for 35 years and has two children: a son, 28, and a daughter, 32. His daughter recently had twin girls. He breaks into a huge smile when he talks about his new granddaughters and his thoughts of playing with them and carrying them on his back as they grow up, just as he did with his own kids. He lives by the motto "health is wealth." It shapes his life's goals, which include time with his children and grandchildren and, as he notes, hopefully great grandchildren. Traveling the world with his wife is also a major goal. He is acutely aware that health is a prerequisite for all that life holds, and has translated these major goals into a series of social and behavioral routines that sustain his lifestyle.

When he describes his approach to healthy living, it becomes clear that Vijay is a creature of habit. His routines are the cornerstone of both his social motivation and behavior. When his children were young, he regularly took his family to India. It was a ritual imbedded in the family culture. So much so, it served as inspiration for his son to pursue a career in public health, after witnessing the conditions in their native country. Today, Vijay and his wife make monthly visits to see their daughter. Initially they went to Miami and now to Iowa, where she has relocated with her husband and those new twin girls. Vijay tells me that he does not want to end up in a nursing home or lose his independence. He enjoys the freedom to work and travel that his health provides.

His behavior is further evidence of his ability to structure day-to-day activities in support of his life's goals and leverage the power routine:

> No, I don't go to any gym because of work. I don't get the time to spend two or three hours in the gym. But, what I do, I keep my routine regularly—so that's even though it's the weekend, holiday, or weekday.

Vijay spells out his rituals for me, which he credits as a major contributor to his health. He wakes up like clockwork every day between 5:30 and 6:00 a.m. is in bed by 9:30 or 10 p.m., and always eats at the same time. At least three times a week, he walks the halls of a nearby shopping mall and extends his exercise, by being sure to walk the stairs. "I wake up regularly, eat my meals regularly, I do the walk in the evening, and make sure I do the steps."

His habits include staying away from processed and greasy foods and soda. He utilizes portion control and tries to eat two or three servings of fruits and vegetables every day. His advice for men is to stay consistent in your daily activities and maintain a regular schedule. "Everything should be regular," he says.

Vijay has internalized his routine and the link to his life's goals. He enjoys his lifestyle and its benefits. If his motto, health is wealth, is true, then Vijay is a very wealthy man.

## Implementing Your Goals: Getting Where You Want to Be

If there is anything I've learned in my 63 years, it's that nothing worthwhile comes easy. If you want robust inspiration, and if you seek continuous motivation that you can turn into healthy behaviors, you need to give it the appropriate thought and consideration. After all, we are talking about those things that you hold most precious, the things you love most dearly, and the ability to be healthy enough to enjoy them! So, how can you create your own rhythm? What will it take to turn those high-level goals and aspirations you identified in the exercises in Chapter 5 into concrete objectives, tasks, and tactics? Here is how.

## Creating Your Own Rhythm

It's now time to turn to you and building your own rhythm. So, let's breakdown the process and show you exactly how to assemble a diversified portfolio of activities that will translate your goals into concrete actions. Here is one approach:

## Confirm Your Goals

You always reserve the right to adjust. Now that I've given you some additional examples of how to think about values, priorities, and implementing tactics, if you have some fresh thoughts about your headline goals, now's the time to adjust, add, or subtract. Will they provide the motivation you need to address any gaps you identified in Chapter 4? Do they truly reflect your priorities? Are they achievable?

At this point, you may want to re-categorize your goals, better define them, or simply restate them in a different way that is more meaningful to you. In addition, you may want to rank-order your goals, so you don't succumb to the very real pitfall of accomplishing a lot of things that hold some value, but less than others. Remember, this whole process is about you feeling comfortable about what you want in life and identifying those activities that will inspire and fulfill your basic needs. This is important. It's not easy. Give it the time and attention it deserves. It's the foundation of the motivational platform and your vehicle to healthy behavior.

## Structure Your Approach

I just introduced you to the social pyramid: my own way of thinking about personal and social activities that tie to my larger goals. I like the approach because it creates diversity, confronts the routine, grind-it-out nature of life, and highlights the need to work proactively on special events. I encourage you consider this model, but there are certainly other ways to think about tailoring your own bundle of activities, based on your individual circumstances. Here are some factors to keep in mind:

### Remember Your Priorities

As I just mentioned, you can, and should, rank-order your goals so your implementing strategies will follow this ranking. These activities have financial, time, and emotional costs. That said, if you're like most of us and don't have unlimited resources, consider your priorities when you plan. If resources are a limitation, the good news is that many social and emotional activities are available through non-monetary events or actions, and many are relatively low in costs. Time spent with loved ones need not break the bank, nor do some of the most basic behavioral activities.

### Fill Up the Year

When contemplating your social agenda, look beyond the next few months. Milestone events will naturally take you into multi-year planning, but at least give some consideration for what you can do during the course of the year. This is where the routine activities really come in handy. If you have family, kids, or grandkids, the fundamentals that come with them go a long way to populating the calendar.

### Diversify

You need to address as many of your goals as possible. If you don't have the time or the ability to act on a goal, park it in the bullpen and call it out only when you can. Listing goals that have no hope of action is a waste of time and simply pulls down your self-administered grade. That said, try to find a variety of approaches toward goal accomplishment. Variety is the spice of life, and there is no reason why you can't experiment with different ways to have fun with your wife and/or kids and hit your mark from divergent angles. Diversity of activity is a cornerstone of my Social Pyramid, so it is high on my list.

### Document Your Outcomes

When I was in a college fraternity, we had a guy who was our designated historian. Translation: he took pictures at all the parties, fundraisers, and sporting events. If it's memories and traditions you're building, then by all means, document them! iPhones and other devices make this easier than ever, although I personally like the idea of displaying an old-fashioned photo as a constant reminder of the special moments.

My dad has been camera crazy since I was born. He actually aspired to be a television cameraman, but his mother told him to be a lawyer, so that's what he did. Nevertheless, I've watched him migrate over the years from the old eight-millimeter camera to video, to Polaroid still shots to today's disposable cameras. Consequently, my entire family and I are on film in one form or another for the past 60+ years. Lesson: It's nice to have the pictures from the big events! By the way, that oldest son I keep mentioning: He received his degree in film from Temple University, and today he and his wife have a successful film company. Guess his grandfather rubbed off on him.

### Consider Other Structures

Maybe the Pyramid doesn't work for you; that's okay. Perhaps a calendar approach is better, organizing your activities based on a daily, weekly, monthly, or annual structure. Alternatively, you can stick with the categories presented in Chapter 5 and anchor your actions around the people and priorities in your life. Any approach that works for you is fine, so long as it has a level of definition and precision where you can measure performance. In the end, it is about doing things that accomplish the goals that produce the motivation that fuels behavior. There is no wrong answer!

### Review for Reasonableness

Finally, I mentioned it above, but it is worth repeating. Make sure that the strategies, objectives, tactics, or actions—whatever you want to call them—are reasonable. Time, money, social conditions, and emotions can all influence your ability to be successful. Don't stretch too far, particularly at the beginning.

The exercise that follows at the end of this chapter provides a grid and sample responses, based on my Social Pyramid. The grid is modifiable to accommodate any approach you choose. What's critical is that you have a structure and organized approach to accomplishing your goals. This is too central to the quality of your life just to wing it. Use exercise and the examples of the last three chapters to strengthen your awareness. Your motivation is right there in front of you, living and breathing in that which you value and hold most precious. Connect the dots, create your rhythm, and enjoy the ride!

## Chapter 6 Exercises

Chapter 6 is about breaking down your goals into specific actions that will enable you to achieve them. To this point, you've given plenty of thought to your life's priorities and the factors that represent your strongest social motivators. You've translated these factors into tangible goals that will reinforce your strengths and close the gaps that you've identified. Now, you need to breakdown these goals into discrete actions that you'll carryout throughout the course of the year. This is how you'll achieve your vison and track performance. These are your behavioral guardrails. They keep you on track.

As a simple step to guide you in the design your own strategies, review the following table. It's an illustration of the Social Pyramid representing the spouse/partner goal categories. When designing your personal strategies, feel free to add additional categories and expand the table to include as many goals as you wish. The more customized the better. Again, this need not be a solo effort. Engage others. Good luck.

## SPOUSE/PARTNER GOALS

| CATEGORY | WEEKLY | MONTHLY | ANNUALLY | COMMENTS |
|---|---|---|---|---|
| **ROUTINE GOALS** | | | | |
| #1 Dinner dates | Dinner together Friday night @ casual, local restaurant. | At least once a month go into the city for a more formal dinner. | Something special at Valentine's Day, and our birthdays. | Get away to chill out and catch up. |
| #2 Movies | Watch a move at home. | Catch a movie at a theater at least one a month. | Try to see as many Oscar-nominated movies. | "On Demand-subscription movies on TV work just as well. |
| #3 Shopping, local sight-seeing | Bolt on a Friday night stroll after your dinner in the nice weather. | Get out and do something together a couple of times a month. | Candlelight shopping at Christmas, Fireworks on July 4th. | This is another great way to share time together w/o any heavy-duty planning. Often spur-of- the-moment. |
| **SPECIAL GOALS** | | | | |
| #1 Attend NFL game together. | N/A | N/A N/A | One or two games per season. | Works while the weather is still warm. |
| #2 Go to New York to see a Broadway show. | N/A | N/A | One or two trips per year. Long weekend. | Love the "Big Apple." Lots of fun. |
| #3 Vacation in Florida or Caribbean. | N/A | N/A | Once a year. | "Chillin'" by the pool is the best. |
| **BONDING GOALS** | | | | |
| #1 Visits from out-of-town family. | N/A | N/A | Organize visit from one or more siblings, usually summer or holidays. | Staying close to those far away is important to us. |

## SPOUSE/PARTNER GOALS (continued)

| CATEGORY | WEEKLY | MONTHLY | ANNUALLY | COMMENTS |
|---|---|---|---|---|
| **BONDING GOALS** | | | | |
| #2 Spend time together with our grandson. | Babysit, grab dinner, or just visit. | Visit a museum or do something together. | Make the most of birthdays, holidays, special occasions. | Spending time with our grandson brings us closer together. |
| #3 Milestone B-Days | | | Out-of-town parties and family gatherings to create special b-day memories. | Celebrated my 60th in Las Vegas w/ siblings and and wife. |
| **MILESTONE GOALS** | | | | |
| #1 Son's Wedding | | | Typically, long-lead item that can produce equally long span of motivation and longer memories. | Lifetime of memories. |
| #2 Dad's 90th B-Day Party | | | Inspiration on multiple levels with long-term impact. | Family and friends, a well-deserved tribute to our dad. |
| #3 Trip to Europe | | | A milestone that drives home the purpose of maintaining your health. | Bonding on several levels; family, fun, and new experiences. |

Figure 10: Spouse/Partner Goals

# 7

## Create Your Personal Lifestyle Network

ONE OF MY MOST consistent findings on 50+ men who maintain a healthy lifestyle is the significance of their relationships. They find inspiration in partnerships that support their behaviors. Whether family, friends, business associates, or others, men who share social interests, health goals, and behaviors with others are more successful in achieving those goals and maintaining healthy behaviors. Thus, for the next strategy I focus on partnerships.

Whether they're working out to be able to maintain caretaking duties for a stricken spouse or training to tackle their grandchildren in preparation for next weekend's visit, men are motivated and sustained in their healthy behaviors by their closest relationships. Almost three-quarters of the men I studied combine their social relationships and their health-related behaviors with a friend, spouse, or other individual. Further, 98% find that doing so is helpful in maintaining their healthy lifestyle.

On the surface, it may seem almost cliché to suggest that partnerships increase the likelihood that men will adopt and maintain healthy behaviors. Sure, it helps to have a gym buddy, but the issue is much deeper and more complex. What I'm suggesting goes way beyond the gym buddy.

In my research, I encountered men who distributed their partnerships across several acquaintances, as well as those who concentrated theirs in a single individual with equal success and satisfaction. Some study participants limited their engagement to a spouse for one specific health behavior, usually diet, or exercise. Others received support from a broader range of their family through a variety of social activities. Then there were men who found great motivation in their friends, often including both social and behavioral dimensions.

Partners come in many shapes and sizes, and your relationships can take many forms, but their involvement is a universal strategy among healthily living men. If you're looking to become healthy, building a good social network and developing the social skills to acquire and retain new partners is foundational.

In this chapter, I'll break down various categories and types of partnerships to give you some deeper insights into how you can maximize the power of partnerships and develop this core element of your lifestyle architecture. In addition, I'll provide stories from two men, each of whom have implemented social supports in different ways and tailored their support systems based on their individual goals and circumstance.

## Models of Partnering Behavior

Let's start with a look at the three main types of partnerships found in my research: social, behavioral, and blended.

Social partnerships are just that, relationships founded on a social connection: a family member, friend, or other socially based affiliation. With families or good friends, an emotional bond is often present, a strong source of motivation. The men value the relationship and build social activities around these interactions: travel with a spouse, time vacationing with children, or grandchildren, or social-izing with friends. The more enduring the social bonds, the stronger the motivation and underlying emotional ties become. The social and emotional benefits of time spent in these relationships energize men. The emotional investment and the resulting motivation fuel their healthy behavior. Social partners can also perform as fans and cheerleaders in support of your health aspiration. If aware of your goals, they can provide welcome encouragement and feedback.

Behavioral partnerships are more functional and tactical. They represent the means through which the healthily-behaving men find support for the daily grind of their lifestyles. They range from the gym buddy and walking partner, to the friend with whom they share a hobby, a recreational sport teammate, or a colleague who shares in healthy cooking and meal planning. Common interests are what build their bond. Their mutual enjoyment of the partnership has the power to ease what might otherwise be tedious tasks and potentially create a degree of pleasure through the socialization.

Blended partnerships represent a combination of social and behavioral: exercising with your spouse, swimming with your grandchildren, eating healthily with your children, or hiking on a trip with family or friends. A number of the men I interviewed maintained blended partnerships that formed the heart of their lifestyle architecture, producing a significant and steady source of their motivation for their behavior.

Within these broad categories, I found subcategories that approach partnership building from different perspectives. I offer them as a tool to spur your thinking about areas in your life that could benefit from a partnership, and launch your effort to recruit individuals with shared interests.

Site-specific partnerships can be social, behavioral, or blended relationships unique to a location, such as home, work, the gym, and are generally restricted to actions and interactions at that location. An example of site-specific partnerships would include work colleagues who support one another in healthy eating habits during lunch or time at an on-site fitness center. Limited to the workplace, this relationship does not persist in after-hours nutritional decision-making. It applies only to behavior sets that occur in the context of the shared space.

You form activity-specific relationships around a common interest in unique actions whether social, behavioral, or blended. Examples include travel, arts, hobbies, diet, exercise, or stress management.

It is important to emphasize that these categories and sub-categories are a means to guide your thinking about needs and sources of relationships that can increase your ability to sustain a healthy lifestyle. While I have constructed distinct categories to encourage thought, it is important to acknowledge that the same individual (i.e., your spouse) may fulfill needs or provide a resource in overlapping categories and extend the blended partnership concept into multiple dimensions. Significant social partners can represent a strong source of motivation, while also representing a behavioral partner that joins you in a number of activity-specific relationships and more. How you design your individual network of partners is up to you. It's a product of your individual needs and interests, and what value you bring to your prospective partners.

## — An All-Points Bulletin —

Jay makes slipcovers. It is a dying industry, as he will readily tell you. At 84, he is self-employed and maintains a client list of faithful and returning customers. His work keeps him engaged and energetic, it stimulates his body and mind, and it helps to structure his day. While his business has shrunk from a peak of 25 employees to a one-man operation, he enjoys the rhythm of the work and the freedom it affords him to travel. His healthy lifestyle began with the medical emergency of a loved one, and the practices seemed to have taken root in his family.

He recounts a story for me as we sit at a conference table in suburban New Jersey, "When I hit 50, my mother had a heart attack; she had three of them." Pausing for a moment, he absentmindedly brushes his eye. "It was a wake-up call for me. I lost 35 pounds in four months. I laid-off the junk. I have a lot of self-control. I'm disciplined."

Smiling, his shoulders move in a self-deprecating shrug, as if to downplay the ease with which he reports the transformation. "My daughter is like me in that respect; my son is more like my wife. He works out three times a week."

When I ask Jay, "Do you share your health behaviors with anyone?" He replied:

> My doctor friend, I'm very close with, for about 35 years. We go out to dinner. We used to play racquetball. He's 79, and he still gets around very well. We go out to dinner, if he orders the salmon, I order the salmon.

Jay has just described a blended partnership. As a close friend and dinner companion, their social connection anchors their relationship. The doctor's support of a healthy diet extends their interaction into Jay's behavior. As we continue, Jay hesitates for a moment:

> My wife, she eats healthy, but she snacks a lot. My daughter really cooks healthy. When we go for dinner, she'll have a roasted chicken or grilled salmon. My wife will eat that, but she still brings in snacks: Oreo cookies.

For a moment, he is clearly uncomfortable, and the conversation has strayed into unfamiliar territory. His wife certainly represents a social partner. She is aware of his goals and broadly supports his behaviors, but, in this case, the relationship does not extend into the blended realm, as she does not participate in those behaviors herself. This stands in contrast to his daughter's role as a site-specific social partner. She provides practical support by preparing healthy meals when Jay visits, but can only support this health behavior in her own home, as she can't follow her parents' home and police their behavior. Indeed, as beneficial as allies prove to be in maintaining health, the question of how to respond to a spouse or significant other who is unwilling or unable to practice a healthy lifestyle figures prominently in my conversations with healthy men.

Jay goes on to confess that he would like to travel, but his wife's health impedes her mobility and willingness to drive or fly, and she has suggested he travel with his sister, with whom he is close. While touched by her desire to see him happy, the lost opportunity to share the experiences of his twilight years with his wife pains him. In spite of excellent health and health behaviors, a long-held goal seems out of reach; while his relationship is strong, an important aspect of this partnership is missing.

Jay is an example of the application of an excellent sustainability trait, multidimensional partnering, by constructing a network of individuals for support and encouragement in different health behaviors. His professional life and relationships stimulate consistent activity, while his friends and children are integral to his nutritional outlook.

Next, we will look at an example of unidimensional partnering, or sharing most behavior sets with a single individual.

## — Good Cop-Better Cop —

John and his wife Mary are both retired. Their children, grown and married with children of their own, live nearby. They spend their days walking, working in their garden, playing with their grandchildren, and relaxing with a book or early matinée. For more than thirty years, the couple maintained a strict vegetarian diet.

Leaning back in his chair John recollects, "My wife became a vegetarian in, what was it, 1982. I was working at the time, and she prepared all of our meals, so that meant that I was a vegetarian as well."

During his long career as a marketing executive, John was the family breadwinner, with Mary running their home and caring for their children. She served as a social partner in a site-specific partnership (by preparing meals at home that met their shared vegetarian standards) and as an activity-specific partner (by encouraging

John to maintain this dietary practice in all meals). After he retired and they found themselves empty nesters with too much time and too little to keep themselves occupied, John awakened to the world of cooking and nutrition.

Describing the evolution of their shared palette in those early years, he admits:

> At first it was something we did to maintain a healthy weight, to stay trim, but we've made some changes over the years. We've tried raw food and paleo diets; we've done our macronutrient counts; now we're strict vegans. Now it's more about keeping ourselves healthy for one another.

Since their adoption of a vegetarian diet, John has become a proficient cook, and they have both become expert gardeners, producing much of their own food during the summer and fall months. Where food preparation was a practical matter intended to support healthy weight, it has become a shared endeavor, in which the couple produces ingredients, plans menus, and prepares their meals together.

John gets a lot of satisfaction from the process, and opines:

> Our garden is a great source of stress-relief. We work together, but there isn't a lot of pressure; it's relaxing. We'll see which vegetables are coming along and get ideas for what to make for dinner; we discuss recipes. There's really nothing like a meal you've produced entirely with your own hands.

At age 72, both he and Mary look younger than their years, and report high energy, as well as optimism regarding their relationship and aging prospects. They cite one another as their most important sources of support and motivation, and they seamlessly trade duties as coach and caretaker, when necessary. John and Mary provide an excellent example of unidimensional partnering, in which one shares most of their health behaviors with a single individual. One may consider this model as your traditional married couple: they know one another intimately, they share daily rhythms and habits, and they are up to speed on one another's health status and goals. The most significant benefit of this mode of partnering is the constant and consistent nature of the relationship. A single individual with whom you interface for a wide range of behaviors is able to assess comprehensively all behaviors and is likely to notice changes in state, energy, and habit. The biggest weakness of this model, of course, is that it puts all your metaphorical eggs in one basket, leaving dramatic implications for men who lose their life partner.

## A Strong Health Network Requires Diverse Partners

Earlier in the book, I introduced the concept of a personal health network, modeled after the much larger, diversified networks of physicians, hospitals, and other providers developed and maintained by health insurers. Both Jay and John exhibit partnering behaviors that support their healthy lifestyle and subsequent outcomes, a trend borne out by the men I surveyed and the bulk of clinical evidence. We know that married men live longer, and experience better health across the board than their single counterparts. The loss of a spouse, either via bereavement or divorce, is associated with negative health outcomes in men who then remain single (men who remarry following the departure of a spouse/companion tend to avoid these negative effects) (Cohen, 2004).

Married men tend to have lower levels of hypertension and a mortality rate 46 percent lower than that of their unmarried peers. Conversely, American, British, and Israeli studies demonstrate that marital turmoil is associated with a roughly 35 percent increase in subject's risk of heart attack, angina, and stroke (Cohen, 2004), while marital satisfaction has been shown to moderate levels of the stress hormone cortisol in both men and women (Saxbe, 2008).

Divorce is also closely associated with an increase in male suicides, though not in female suicides. Although studies show that marriage does not alter the incidence of cancer, it correlates with increased survival time in individuals diagnosed with cancer, and unmarried individuals are more likely to receive their diagnoses in later stages of the disease. In comparing rates of prostate cancer survival, married men averaged 69 months following their diagnoses, men who had never married averaged 49 months, and separated or widowed men averaged 38 months (Saxbe, 2008)

You'd think that these statistics might spell disaster for single, divorced, and widowed men, or suggest that the only possible salvation for their health is to marry, and fast. I would argue that a more optimistic mechanism for healthy partnering is available regardless of your relationship status. Men who successfully team up in support of their health recognize a diverse array of potential supporters, and cultivate support for their habits wherever available. They do not surrender to a solitary struggle in the face of lost support, whether due to death, disability, or disinclination.

Jay and John rely on partnerships that are distinctly different, yet equally valid, Jay with his children and friends, John with his wife. Each receives motivational and substantive support from their chosen health partners; both report increases in positive dietary behaviors and activity levels achieved with the support of friends and loved ones. The most important behavior that my participants impart is that they share their behaviors. They do not attempt to achieve their goals alone, but instead recruit their supporters as cheerleaders and coaches.

What I've shown in my survey of 1,000 healthy men and in these case studies is that partnering works! You can increase your chances of adopting and maintaining a healthy lifestyle if you reject going it alone, recognize your strengths and weaknesses, and look for teammates who can help you fill the gaps. As we've seen, companions come in all forms, from family, to friends, to professional relationships. Married or single, you can find someone to meet your needs. Partners are available in any number of places from your social network to professional, religious, and civic organizations in which you may participate. And, they can range from one or two to several, depending on your circumstances. As a model, think of your support team as the health insurers think about their provider networks. Set up your own network of health-supporting allies, based on where and when you need a boost. By approaching your goal of healthy behavior in this fashion, you'll be one-step ahead of the game and on your road to success.

# Chapter 7 Exercises

Chapter 7 is about the power of partnerships and creating your own support network. The process of building a group of family members, friends, and colleagues can be fun and mutually beneficial to you and your recruits. Their role can be social or behavioral (i.e., diet and exercise). Your simple step in this action is to consider the following questions. Built off the categories in the chapter, they will help you develop your own network. As you reflect on the questions, you'll no-doubt get some ideas as to how you can also grow your own social skills. How would you answer the following questions?

## Warm-up Drill:
## Identifying Individuals for Your Network

- Can you identify individuals who share your interest in a robust social life?
- Do any of these same people aspire to lead a healthy lifestyle?
- Have you ever discussed your personal priorities with anyone and the motivation it brings to live healthily?

- Have you thought about those aspects of your lifestyle (social or behavioral) where having the support of a friend or colleague would provide a boost?
- What can you offer to others who aspire to live healthily?

## Mapping Your Assets

- Can you name five individuals who you'd like to make part of your healthy behavior support network?
- Do you have a specified role for each?
- Is there something that they need which you can provide?
- Do your network partners address all the gaps in your lifestyle architecture that you've identified?

## Implementing Your Network

- How can you best share your story of social motivators and goals for a healthy lifestyle with each network member?
- How did they react to your story?
- Have you offered your support to these individuals?
- How does your network break down between social and behavioral partners?
- What exactly are your partners "bringing to the table?"

## Work Your Partnerships

- Are your partnerships working?
- Do they provide the support you need to overcome the hurdles you identified?
- Do your partners believe that your support of them is making a difference?
- Are you having fun?

## Evaluate and Adjust

- Are you tracking your partner relationships?
- Are you happy with the outcomes so far?
- Do you feel the need to change any of your partners?
- If asked, what would your partners say about you?
- Are you prepared to seek new partners in certain areas, if necessary?

# 8

# Design a Sustainability Plan

SUSTAINABILITY IS A HOT concept today that is most frequently associated with policies and practices concerning the environment. At its core, however, sustainability is about the endurance of systems and processes, and that's the connection to our discussion of motivation and behavior. For us, sustainability means tailoring a lifestyle with your own customized systems and processes that you can maintain over the long haul: think behavioral longevity.

Yes, it is critical to start the journey by assessing your current behaviors. Certainly, you need to identify your personal goals. Day to day, it's important to get into a rhythm, where your motivations and behaviors flow in a synchronized fashion. That said, what's essential, what's most critical, and what the healthy guys demonstrate is sustainability: the ability to navigate the trials and tribulations that life throws at you and still maintain the motivation and behavior over time.

As in many things in life, getting there is one thing, but staying there is another thing entirely. A sustainability plan takes your game to the next level. It strengthens the fabric of your social model, forming a safety net that keeps you in rhythm when times get tough and threaten your positive behavior patterns. It's preparedness on a personal basis.

## The Sustainability Continuum

The Sustainability Continuum is the conceptual framework I've labeled to encompass a collection of strategies designed to enhance behavioral longevity. The name reflects my vision of a progressive set of tactics that promote self-organization, reinforcement of positive behavior, the application of strategy, and best practices from the field of psychology. The continuum has four pillars: acknowledgement, fortification, rejuvenation, and invention. Together, they represent the architecture within which you can customize the engineering of your behaviors for endurance.

## Acknowledgment: There Will Be Potholes Along the Journey

Fundamental to building a strategy for sustainability is acknowledging that there will be potholes along your journey. You need to be prepared. It is naïve to think that maintaining healthy living is easy. It's not. Recognizing the depth and dimensions of the impediments you will encounter is smart. Major league sports teams spend millions scouting their opponents and then sizing up their strengths and weaknesses before each game. Their experts look for every nuance in the opponent that may give them an edge to use, and these reports help to shape their game plans when they meet on the field. They know what to expect and are prepared with a strategy to counter their opponent.

When it comes to your life: your priorities, strengths, weaknesses, and abilities, you're the expert. With the possible exception of your wife or significant other, you know yourself better than anyone else does. If you're honest, your insights can go a long way to building your game plan for sustaining healthy behavior. Let's go deeper, so there's no misunderstanding.

Even if you've successfully thought through your values, identified your personal priorities, established motivation-generating social goals, and embarked on a series of routines that have created a rhythm in your life, stuff happens. We all fall off the horse of motivation and healthy behavior; we become disrupted by family issues, business distractions, and personal dilemmas. We invert our values. Trivial matters attract undue attention, leaving true priorities twisting in the wind. However, as Rocky Balboa once said, "It ain't about how hard ya hit. It's about how hard you can get hit and keep moving forward," (Stallone, 2017). Be prepared for the hits.

The good news is that my research suggests that healthy behaviors stick; 74% of the men I surveyed have been living a healthy lifestyle for 11 years or more. Men 70 and over are more likely to have been living a healthy lifestyle for years longer than their younger cohorts, indicating that the lifestyle is certainly attainable and sustainable into upper age ranges. The healthy guys find a way to sustain their behaviors. They work through the hits and stay on track. So can you.

## Fortification: Keep Your Values Front & Center

So, what exactly does it mean to be prepared? How do healthy males stay focused and on track? How do they fortify their motivations and behaviors to weather the tough times? For starters, the research suggests that the men keep their values front and center. As you'll remember, when asked, 74% said that they think about their priorities quite often. Therefore, one of the first strategies is keeping your values on top of your mind. How do you do this? Here's one approach.

### The Speech Strategy

Have you ever had to give a speech or a brief talk? Maybe you had a quick huddle of friends or co-workers, where people are looking to you for your thoughts? One example is the elevator speech. You quickly summarize your attributes, should you step on an elevator with that executive you've been trying to reach for your job search. If you've experienced any of this, you know that it helps to be prepared. You're much more effective if you've thought about the message, the audience, and the key points you need to make to evoke the action you want from those listening. Whether you use bullet points or a fully written speech, the exercise requires some thought and reflection, not to mention the substantive accomplishments and achievements that form the content of your speech.

Now suppose you had to deliver a speech about your life: your values, priorities, and, most importantly, what you were doing that day, that month, or that year that propelled you to act on those priorities. What would you say? What stories could you tell? How passionately would you deliver the message? Would there be emotion in your voice? Would you come across as sincere and committed to your values?

If you'd have plenty to say, with specific illustrations that support your major goals in life, then chances are that you're likely on a path to sustainable behavior and good health. The availability of substantive content and a passionate delivery suggests that you are carrying out your life's goals and generating a wellspring of motivation. If you'd have to really think about it, and scramble to assemble a decent list of actions you've taken, then I'd say your "sustainability quotient" is on the low side. Either way, understand that you need to keep your values at the forefront of your mind if you're going to maintain your lifestyle through the bumps. When your values represent the underpinnings of your motivation and behavior, then you benefit from fortifying these factors as much as possible, to build the behavioral strength to endure the challenges you'll no doubt face.

A speech also offers a great metaphor for the mechanics of motivational and behavioral fortification. Planning a speech requires you to re-think your goals for consistency and practicality with your life circumstances. Are you making sense to the audience? Do the tactics and strategies align with your priorities? Is your presentation compelling? Are you in a position to update your speech over time? Are you able reflect on wonderful memories of accomplishments, as well as describe plans for future activities with family or friends?

Try this out. Hold your own private briefing every Friday at 5 p.m. You're the CEO of your life, and it's time for your weekly press conference with yourself. What's your message? What did you do this week to carry out your goals? What were your successes and shortcomings? How does next week look? I find that a weekly recap is a great way to both celebrate the week's achievements and challenge myself on the unfinished business. My agenda is wide ranging and includes everything from scheduling the plumber, making a date with my wife, time with our new grandson, an important business meeting, and my daily workouts. It's about using the systems and processes of my life to stay focused and on track.

The speech metaphor has another important dimension to sustaining behavior, and that is the commitment. As a psychological exercise, pretend you're in a position of power, an elected official perhaps. Further, pretend that you are giving a speech that includes a series of commitments to take certain actions or pursue a particular course of action. The expectation is that the audience and others will hold you accountable for those commitments, and, consequently, you'll take them seriously and work hard to not to break what some might say are the promises you made in the speech. Now, just like we did earlier, suppose that your speech is one that you are giving, and it's about the commitments that you've made to yourself and your loved ones. How would you feel? Would you take those commitments just a little more seriously? What if your speech was about your life and you made it to friends or others to whom you were close? Would your expanding audience heighten your awareness of these commitments and increase your motivation to make good on them? I think it would. Some may see this as a matter of pride or a desire not to fail. Others may simply utilize this exercise to remain aware of their priorities—to keep them front and center when there are competing factors for your attention. Either way, talking about your values and goals—whether to yourself or others—represents a commitment, a commitment that you reinforce every time you make that speech. It can be a great tool to help keep your priorities central and fortify your motivations and behaviors.

## Rejuvenation

Rebounding is an important skill in basketball. It's accepted that players won't make every shot, so the ability to "control the boards" (i.e., rebound well) is integral to success. This is true in life as well. You're not going to make 100% of your shots, so accept the premise and acknowledge the importance of bouncing back from miscues. The healthy guys do it. Of the men I surveyed, 43% said that they maintain a contingency plan when they can't exercise or engage in their hobby as scheduled. Anecdotally, many of the men I interviewed found that the absence of an installment in their exercise routines or hobbies produced a level of discomfort, remedied only by a return to the healthy activity. Rejuvenation is as much a part of a healthy lifestyle as any other element. When you designed your lifestyle architecture to minimize any departure from your social and behavioral routines, when it inevitably happens, be prepared to rebound, or get back on the horse of life and press on. What's the mindset required to accomplish this?

One perspective that can help is to go back to basics and consider the underlying motivations that got you started on your journey: your priorities. My guess is that most, if not all, of your most highly valued priorities in life are still there as a source of inspiration. When I asked my study group, 98% said that the same factors that caused them to start living healthily are the ones that still motivate them to maintain their lifestyles. The results were the same across all age groups. If some of your priorities are gone, then there are others waiting for discovery in other parts of your life. If you were able to construct a social-personal-motivational-behavioral relationship, then you have the ability to reactivate it as a means to rejuvenate your beneficial behavior, if you've strayed from your lifestyle. This is doable on your own through simple reflection, through conversations, calls, visits, or even technology (i.e., Skype visits with the kids or grandkids). Whatever it takes to remind yourself of what you have to live for, and what is most important in your life, is an acceptable strategy for rejuvenation.

Many years ago, I used this tactic successfully, albeit in a professional setting. While it didn't concern my commitment to healthy living, it is very much analogous because it was all about rejuvenation and motivation. I served as a county administrator in my early 30s and, while I loved my job, I was not immune to the pressures of the position. The responsibilities of managing a $200 million county government and the overlaying politics would occasionally diminish my enthusiasm. In those instances, I employed a very simple strategy that quickly brought back my inspiration and enthusiasm. I visited the senior day care center, or perhaps some other social service we operated. It was the perfect antidote. Seeing the seniors working on their arts and crafts, enjoying each other's company, and just generally having fun brought me back to this core mission of the county and how we affected people's lives for the good. It was my own version of the "management by walking around," theory from back in the day (Peters & Waterman, 1982).

This really was a restorative and therapeutic exercise, and it immediately restored my motivation to get back to my office and tackle what the day had in store. The factors that had diminished my enthusiasm suddenly didn't appear to be so troubling.

For men whose enthusiasm for healthy behavior diminished for any reason, for those that life has thrown some curveballs, find your own rejuvenation process, just as I found mine as a young man. In the psychology literature, this is cognitive reframing, and its effects are very beneficial (Beck, 1997). It can be as simple as a call to your children. Maybe it's a trip. Whatever it takes, the simple message from our healthy men is to have a contingency plan. Recognize the difficulty embedded in the search for sustainability and prepare accordingly.

## Invention

Necessity is the mother of invention, and your health is more necessary than anything else, particularly as you age. Accordingly, invention gets a seat at the table of sustainability as the fourth and final pillar. The men that I've studied are clear and consistent. Motivation is a very personal and individual phenomenon that you can modify and tailor to your meet your changing needs. Whether you need an inventive approach to restart your healthy behavior, or you simply want to grow your motivational portfolio for added security, potential sources of encouragement surround you. Use them. Not only will they strengthen your ability to sustain your healthy behaviors, you'll get the added benefit of social and personal rewards as well.

Expanding the depth and dimensions of your macro social relationships such as wives, children, or grandchildren is a great place to start. Microfactors like garage hobbies, yardwork, or ballgames are all possibilities. An important business meeting, the day's to-do list, or the next 5K race can all be catalysts that you may not currently employ in your thinking.

No matter what your age, there are no hard and fast rules about growing your motivational and behavioral infrastructure. It need not, and should not, be a static process. Motivation and the ability to turn motivation into healthy behavior are wide open for creativity and innovation. My survey data certainly portrays the healthy men as an inventive bunch. Among men that employ habits and rituals, we see a number of creative rituals that received high rankings:

- Building exercise or physical activity into vacations or business trips: 61%.

- Using exercise or your hobby as time to reflect on personal or work-related issues: 52%.

Combining innovation with fortification—keeping your values top of mind—forms a strong motivational and behavioral safety net that will help you increase your potential to continue your healthy behaviors. As you will read in the following case studies of men facing incredibly tough challenges to their behavior, inventive strategies work. They can strengthen your social-behavioral fabric to enable you to meet the tests you'll face head on and succeed.

The bottom line: What you do to stay motivated and engaged doesn't matter nearly as much as having your own set of guardrails to help keep you on track. They can change, evolve, or modify endlessly to suit your needs. Here are two examples of men who have sustained their healthy lifestyles despite significant threats. Both men have persevered in their healthy behaviors by staying anchored to their core motivations and by building innovative approaches to meet what life has presented to them.

## — The Diplomat —

Kevin is 53. He married at 39 and has three children: two boys ages 12, 10, and a girl who is eight. A musician and entertainment entrepreneur, he often works nights and weekends. Since he was a kid, Kevin has been athletic and active in sports. Despite the challenges of a family and a job that has him out many nights a week, Kevin runs three to four days a week, works out at home, and plays in both basketball and baseball leagues. His boys are on the local swim team, so he swims every summer as well. Outdoor trips, skiing in Vermont, fresh air, and the beach are his travel preferences.

He eats whole grain cereals in the morning and salads at lunch. Organic peanut butter, hummus, and blue corn chips fill the gaps. He tries to eat organically as much as possible. Kevin tries to stay away from red meat, choosing organic chicken as an alternative. Soy, almond, and coconut milk are also staples of his diet. He credits his interest in nutrition to a roommate and nutrition courses in college. He even has his 12-year-old son drinking aloe vera juice to help his athletic performance.

Kevin's focus is clearly on healthy living. His advice for 50+ men who want to live healthily is discipline. "You know, a successful businessman stays focused. He's disciplined on accomplishing that goal. It's no different in maintaining a healthy lifestyle."

What makes Kevin's story particularly interesting and a case study in sustainability, is the way he manages his relationship with his wife. When I asked Kevin if his wife shares his healthy lifestyle, the answer without hesitation is no. "She's not against it," he says. "It's a lifelong education campaign because she comes from a meat and potatoes family background—she's just starting to read labels on products."

When I ask Kevin how he handles this difference in their orientation to nutrition day to day he is candid, indicating that sometimes there is a conflict, but one that he's able to manage with the skill of a United Nations diplomat:

> "I say, 'No thank you', if it's a meal that's heavy and thick in cheese, for instance, which is bad for cholesterol, or red meats. I just say 'No, thank you'. And then there are other times, just to keep the peace, I'll have a little bit."

What's even more interesting, and a tribute to Kevin's commitment to sustaining both his marriage and his healthy lifestyle, is the family's shopping habits:

> "We both do food shopping. I'll do my food shopping—and hope that she uses as many of the products and vegetables and fruits that I shop for, because it's going to be the healthiest choices. She does her own shopping because she likes meat."

A vegetable garden enables Kevin to combine his social activities with his healthy living, by engaging his children in the garden:

> "I teach my kids about, you know, how to grow and tend to a vegetable garden. The kids enjoy that. They like to see a plant grow from a seedling and see vegetables and the fruit that it bears. And they enjoy seeing it ripen, and then going out to pick it, and then showing Mommy and Daddy, this is what I grew."

Their excitement provides Kevin with a lot of satisfaction on many levels. The experience contributes to his drive and enables him to balance his family with his healthy values.

What are Kevin's final words of advice for his 50+ brothers? "I think there's always hope for people that are out of shape and want to try to get in shape and live a healthy lifestyle. There's always hope in people; they can do it."

## — A Huge Pothole —

Robert is a 62-year-old widower originally from Tennessee with a 29-year-old daughter who lives with him. He is a human resources executive, currently between jobs. As a boy, he spent time in Okinawa. His father was in the Air Force, so he and his family experienced different cultures, which he cites as an influence on his spiritual and physical philosophy. His wife passed away in 2013 after a period of long illness. They were married for about 27 years. Robert cared for her while she was ill for about two years. While generally healthy, Robert has a predisposition towards high blood pressure and has to watch his cholesterol.

Monday through Friday, he does some form of exercise at home, whether it is calisthenics, lifting weights, stretching, or aerobic exercises. He alternates his routine every other day. He walks his dog twice a day, trying to incorporate even more activity into his daily routine. Robert's healthy behaviors go back to his college days, and perhaps even before. He believes he is self-motivated. During his interview, he says, "I don't need external motivators to do what I need to do."

Robert doesn't use salt; he reads labels and only uses sugar in his coffee. He eats a lot of salads and fruit and tries to drink a lot of water. Over the past few years, Robert focused more intently on his spirituality and religious beliefs. Professionally, he believes that his healthy lifestyle helps him to keep up with the younger men and women in what is a very competitive industry.

Robert's healthy lifestyle was a major factor in his ability to care for his wife and sustain his behaviors throughout her illness:

> I think if I would have been any other—in any other perspective or frame of mind it would have—I would have not been able to support her as well as I tried to support her, because I would have needed help myself, you know. And that would have been a down spiral for both of us.

The strength of Robert's commitment to healthy living is also evident in his relationship with his daughter, a relationship that presents additional challenges to his behaviors:

> Well, my daughter, she—she's—she has some challenges. Put it that way. She has some challenges that she's dealing with. I'm trying to help her as best as I can, you know, trying to enroll other entities to help her. As far as—so there's not really a strong connection there with, you know, her believing the same thing I believe or, you know, expressing the same emotions that I may show in regards to certain topics.

## Sustainability

Kevin and Robert have sustained their healthy behavior through some very difficult situations that may have derailed the rhythm of other men. To their credit, they have fortified their commitment with a focus on their priorities and used inventive strategies to manage day to day. Kevin remains inspired by his family to remain active and overcome a difficult work schedule and a difference in dietary values between him and his wife. Robert ties his ability to sustain a healthy regimen throughout his wife's illness and now his daughter's challenges, to his faith. In both cases, they've acknowledged the confrontations they face, remained focused on their priorities, and used inventive approaches to stay on course without suspending their behavior. They are champions of sustainable behavior!

## Sustainability: Insights from the Field of Psychology

If you are serious about maintaining your behavior over the long haul, you'll be happy to know that behavioral psychologists have examined the conditions that foster sustainable behavior. Here's one illustration that provides some context for our conversation.

Previously, I introduced you to Dr. Edward Deci and his ground-breaking work in motivation, Self-Determination Theory (SDT). Our discussion of sustainability warrants another brief reference to SDT and reinforcement of some of its core concepts, as they link so directly to behavioral longevity.

A central premise of SDT is that sustainable behavior and intrinsic motivators link much more closely than extrinsic motivators do. Among the ideas put forth by Deci and Ryan (1985) is the concept of autonomous self-regulation, which encompasses intrinsic motivation (motivation due to the inherent enjoyment derived from the behavior itself), integrated regulation (engagement in behaviors which are congruent with other central personal goals and values), and identi-fied regulation (motivation reflecting the personal value of behavioral outcomes).

Deci and other behaviorists believe that intrinsic motivators are more likely when three basic psychological needs, what they call "psychological nutriments" (Deci & Ryan, 1985), are satisfied. These are autonomy, competence, and relatedness. Autonomy is an under-standing that you are the origin of your behavior, not some external source. Competence is a feeling of being effective. Relatedness is feeling understood by others. According to these experts, contextual and personal factors, optimize such satisfaction for health. (Niemiec, Ryan & Deci, 2009).

Translated, what the behavioral psychologists mean is that you're more likely to stick with your healthy behavior if these needs are satisfied and, consequently, you're more likely to fall within the umbrella of autonomous self-regulation and the more intrinsically based motivations.

Robert and Kevin are successful in maintaining their behaviors in the face of adversity because they ground their behaviors within autonomous self-regulation. Kevin has fun playing basketball and baseball at age 53, so he's well entrenched in the intrinsic category. Likewise, when asked, Robert says flat-out, "I don't need external motivators to do what I need to do—it just makes sense to try to be healthy as you can be."

Behaviorists would likely classify Robert as clearly in the camp of autonomous self-regulation. In sum, both Robert and Kevin have adopted the behaviors by their own choice and have personalized their pathways to enjoy the feeling of healthy living. They have demonstrated their ability to overcome challenges and feel respected and understood.

What does this mean for you? How does all this psychology break down for a guy just trying to stay the healthy course? What this reconciliation with SDT suggests is that there are alternative forms of motivation. The likelihood of sustaining your healthy behavior and enduring that behavior as life's challenges hit you depends greatly by the source of your motivation. What SDT tells us is that the closer you are to those intrinsic motivators, the more anchored your behavior, and, by extension, the more durable your behavior under assault.

The strategies contained in my Continuum of Sustainability emerge from the social and personal factors exhibited by the men who I have studied. They are rooted in the intrinsic life aspirations cited by the experts as central to behavioral longevity. Keep this in mind as you weave your own personal safety net and personal preparedness plan. It is best to achieve sustainability through a foundation made up of your values, priorities, and aspirations.

The following exercise guides you in developing your own sustainability plan, so, when an obstacle hits you, you'll keep moving forward!

# Chapter 8 Exercises

Chapter 8 is about sustaining your healthy behavior by proactively recognizing that occasionally the normal circumstances of life can derail you. It's preparedness on a personal basis. This simple step exercise presents three categories of questions drawn from the Continuum of Sustainability presented in this chapter to guide you in building your own sustainability plan.

## STEP 1: ASSESS YOUR VULNERABILITIES

The planning process starts with a candid assessment of your vulnerabilities, *both social and behavioral.* Your goal is to practice healthy living 24/7, 365 days a year, year in, and year out. A sustainability plan can help you achieve this goal, AND position yourself, should you ever miss a beat in the rhythm of your behavior.

To begin, ask yourself the following questions. Here's a tip: Use your answers from the previous exercises as a reference, so that your sustainability plan is consistent with your gap analysis, goals, and implementation strategies. Areas previously identified as gaps in strengths represent targets for this vulnerability review.

### Social/Personal Vulnerability Questions

- What are my weakest social/personal relationships? Why?

- What social/personal relationships are the least fulfilling? Why?

- What social/personal relationship(s) would I most like to improve?

- What social/personal goals have I yet to achieve? Why?

- What social/personal factors intrude the most into my ability to achieve my goals?

- What interpersonal skills would I like to improve?

- Are there any other areas that I have previously targeted as gaps in my social motivators?

## Behavioral Vulnerability Questions

- What behaviors, routines, or rituals do I least enjoy?

- Which behaviors do I find most difficult to maintain? Why?

- Have I ever stopped or suspended my healthy behavior?
  - If yes, what were the circumstances?
  - What strategies did I use to restart my healthy behavior?

- What are my habits, routines, and rituals? How strong are they in maintaining my behavior?

- Can I count on my lifestyle partners for help to restart my healthy behavior?

---

## STEP 2: TARGET YOUR GAPS

---

Shoring up your weaknesses is job one. Consider the following:

1. What are the top five areas (social/personal and behavioral) where you believe that you are most vulnerable and need to develop strategies to make them strengths?

2. How can you can successfully invert them to become areas
of strength? Remember, you can use strategies that combine
social/personal factors with behavioral tactics (i.e., Kevin's
use of a vegetable garden to grow healthy food, while
simultaneously bonding with his children and teaching
them about healthy living). These dual-purpose strategies
can pay great dividends, while strengthening your healthy
behavior quotient.

---

## STEP 3: HIGHLIGHT YOUR STRENGTHS

---

You can generate some self-support by making an inventory of
the social and behavioral factors that are your strongest and contribute most to your healthy lifestyle. Doing so can inspire further
self-development and strengthen your social-behavioral matrix. Ask
yourself the following:

1. What are my strongest social motivators and relationships?

2. What's behind this strength?

3. How do I maintain these relationships?

4. What tactics from these stronger relationships can I apply
to my areas of weakness?

After you've considered these questions, apply the same questions
to your behavioral strengths, identify your successful tactics, and use
them to plug gaps. You'll be surprised at the great ideas that will flow
from this process.

You're now ready to design your sustainability plan. From the
questions posed in the previous exercises, you already have insights
into your personal motivational goals (i.e., your lifestyle architecture)
and the more detailed implementation strategies (i.e., your lifestyle

engineering). Your sustainability plan becomes an overlay for these core plans. By that, I mean that the sustainability plan reinforces certain targeted areas of your core plan that you have deemed in need of strengthening—either because of potential vulnerability or because of your strengths and the potential to yield more benefits from that strength. Think of it as a plan "update" and make the appropriate changes to your performance scorecard. Use the top five vulnerabilities from your Step 1 assessment to form the core of your plan.

Once you've established your sustainability plan, it's good practice to periodically assess its performance, and determine if the tactics are working or need revision. Remember, it's your plan. You reserve the right to change, alter, or scrap the plan. Good luck.

# 9

# Leverage Micromotivators

YOU BUILD A CHAMPIONSHIP season one game at a time. Great players know it, and great teams follow this mantra. They devise training rituals where they leave no detail unattended and no subtlety is unimportant. Every ounce of effort goes into the day-to-day regimens, practices, and preparations necessary to achieve their goals, as they move through each opponent on their schedule. Healthy living is very much the same. Every day presents new challenges and opportunities to make an installment in your lifestyle, working at your goals one day at a time. Just like the champions, you don't want to overlook the details. As you face your daily battles against the opponents of healthy living, you'll want to find an edge, a means to get a leg-up on your opponents. No matter how small or subtle, the more inspiration and support the better. It can make a big difference.

So far, I have provided you with a new approach to your health and well-being, one based on motivation and the wellspring of inspiration found in your values and life priorities. Steered by the opinions and interviews of more than 1,000 healthy men over age 50, I have walked you through the intersection of motivation and behavior and shown you how men, just like you, have designed lifestyles that bring the two together to form a platform for behavioral longevity. In our journey to healthy living thus far, we traveled through the 10 strategies gleaned from these men, and our discussion has progressed from broad topics such as goal setting and implementation to more narrow areas. Now it's time that I provide you with some more advanced and nuanced thoughts on motivation. To this end, I'll share my own feelings and experiences on the day-to-day support systems I've used for more than a decade to stay on track. So, let's take our conversation to the next level.

## Micromotivators

Micromotivators is the term I use to describe those very granular strategies, feelings, and approaches that can help you carry out your healthy lifestyle day-in and day-out. They are the psychological equivalent of the ligaments that connect your bones. In the motivational context, they connect your macrogoals and ambitions—your lifestyle architecture—with the day-to-day activities necessary to achieve those goals and institutionalize behavior.

Micromotivators are very personal, nuanced, and maybe even a bit silly, but they represent an important element of your social and behavioral infrastructure. My own experience demonstrates that there are ample opportunities where a little mental push or a pro-active approach to overcoming the rigors of daily life can go a long way to supporting the consistent achievement of your ambitions. The men I've interviewed further substantiate their value. In a word, micromotivators are important. They can turn drudgery into opportunity and pain into gain. Dreaded actions can become welcome undertakings. Here's what I mean.

## My Micros

For me, micromotivators are a mainstay of my lifestyle. Beyond the huge impact that they have on my ability to stay consistent with fitness and diet, the micros contribute to my social and professional well-being. This is no small thing. Their contribution to my personal motivation is significant. My morning routine exemplifies the point.

## My Morning Ritual

Weekdays, I follow a three-stage regimen. Together, they make the mornings something to which I look forward and get my day off to a great start. The rituals neutralize stress, promote focus, and generate creativity. Most importantly, they anchor consistency and generate resilience against the forces of defeat.

Its starts with the thought of a great cup of coffee at 4 a.m. and the feeling of solitude that allows me to contemplate my day; I make my to-do list and glance at the headlines in between shaving and dressing for the gym. For some reason, the coffee tastes extra good at that hour. Talk about microfactors! More importantly, this special, very personal time enables me to put in perspective both the day behind and the day ahead, no matter how bad or good and reconcile the immediate state of affairs with the longer-term view. Amazing, that a simple cup of coffee and some quiet time have become so meaningful. This micromotivator has turned the agony of an early rise into one of my life's little pleasures.

I leverage the micros again when I hit the gym. Here, I'll typically pull from an inventory of topics that help drive me to complete the last five minutes on the treadmill, the final set of sit-ups, or the bench press reps. My thoughts typically go to an event on the calendar or within close proximity where I want to excel. Alternatively, I'll focus on a social event of interest. A presentation at work, a social engagement, a family event, or even the anticipated delivery of a purchase can serve as the day's motivational installment, not to mention the good feeling, physically, of completing the exercise. Either way, it's a focal point to link the physical task at hand. Complete the run and I'll deliver a kick-ass presentation. One more crunch and I'll be feeling good at the party. You get it. No need for unique or earth-shattering subject matter, just the strategic use of some very personal and immediate factors, all of which have the ability to deliver a short-term jolt of inspiration.

Finally, it is breakfast time and another look at the papers before I shower and head to work. Who would think that oatmeal could be so inspiring? Call me crazy, but I love my routine. The cup of oatmeal and morning news is another part of my motivational morning, where I've stimulated my mind and body as I prepare for the day. So, add the oatmeal-newspaper step to the inventory of my micromotivators.

The micros continue throughout the day.

## Lunch

My body clock seems to keep perfect time, so, by noon, I am more than ready for lunch, even if I've had to rely on a mid-morning snack of yogurt or a nutrition bar. So, what's my lunch like? Is there a micro-motivator in play? In short, yes. Here's the backdrop.

As a health care executive, my day fills up with meetings, paperwork, and the notorious email in-basket that never seems to fully empty. That said, when I'm not engaged in a luncheon meeting, I use the time to take a breath, finish any papers that I didn't get to at breakfast, and generally clear my head for a nanosecond. This respite in my day allows me the time to utilize my core principles of diet and nutrition. Combined with my access to some decent nutritional resources, this awareness is enough to sustain my focus through lunch and to use my entrée to contribute to my healthy lifestyle. In my case, I'm again fortunate in that I've got a hospital cafeteria (updated with good food, believe it or not) that serves a reasonably good selection of healthy entrées with vegetables and other selections that enable me to stay true to my dietary goals. Looking at the vegetables behind the glass and reading the nutritional signage on display are motivators that reinforce my behavioral guardrails.

So, my microstrategy is simply to leverage the break as a reminder of the larger lifestyle commitment I've made to myself, to practice what I preach as an individual in the health care industry, and to make an installment toward my larger goals by considering the dietary data as the currency that gets deposited into my healthy living account.

## Dinner

Nuts. No, I'm not referring to my choices in life, my wife (love you, honey), or one of my work colleagues. Rather, I'm talking about the microtactic that I use at dinner many nights. See, for me, dinner is a wild card. I'm not always sure what time I'll finish work. I may have a dinner meeting, may be teaching a class, or may be on my own as my wife has her own active lifestyle. What I do know is that by the time I get home, I'm often dead tired and usually famished. That said, whether I'm picking up takeout or having a home-cooked meal I have to resist the temptation to go overboard, particularly when bedtime is not that far away. So, how do I manage? What seems to complement my meal and fill that last crevice of my stomach while giving me the satisfaction, inspiration, and discipline I need to close out dinner in an appropriate fashion? Nuts, typically cashews or almonds, and, for whatever reason, it works for me and makes me feel good. Now, I'm certainly no nutritionist, but I believe that there's a lot worse I could do, and if the nuts alleviate any craving for dessert, then all the better.

So, there you have it. A day in my life, as viewed from the prism of micromotivators, the little nuances, and the tactics that I use to stay within the guardrails of my healthy lifestyle. Quirky? Yes. Maybe a little odd? Certainly. The bottom line is that it works for me. It gets me out of bed at 4 a.m. five days a week, pushes me at the gym, keeps my diet on track, and prevents me from going overboard with a meal when I'm not far from hitting the sack. By the way, I carry this mindset with me when I'm traveling for business or on vacation. I've spent many early mornings in the hotel lobby with my coffee before I head to the gym and then to breakfast for some oatmeal. When you have come to love your routine, it travels well.

Now, let's look at just a few of examples from the men illustrating their use of micromotivators.

### — Tom —

Tom is a very active 78-year-old who has been married for 33 years and has three daughters and three grandchildren. Although diagnosed with prostate cancer many years ago, he is fine today. He is also diabetic, which he manages by taking medicine and watching his diet. Neither of these factors prevents Tom from living an extremely active lifestyle, including hitting the gym two or three days a week, and using the stationary bike, rowing machine, and treadmill, he has at home. Tom's micromotivator is list-making. Besides keeping his busy life straight, daily list-making provides tangible evidence of his social and behavioral activities and reinforces their positive impact on his life. Compiling lists makes Tom feel good:

> I'm a great list-maker. Every morning, every evening, whenever I feel I need to, I make a list. And, I want to accomplish those things that are on the list. It's not a bucket list. It's just things that need to be done that I want to do, and I try to organize so that I get those things done —it just keeps me going. There's always something to do.

### — Harris —

Harris is a 53-year old insurance broker, who is 11 years into his second marriage. He has two older sons from his first marriage and a nine-year-old daughter with his current wife. Harris believes in the principle behind the micromotivators. "For the average person, you have to get them to find something that gets them out of bed every day or something that—that makes them smile, you know, something simple."

In Harris' case, his daily contact with his nine-year-old daughter does the trick. "Maybe just seeing my daughter every day motivates me."

## — Tim —

Tim is 52 and on his second marriage. He has four children: an adult son and daughter from his first marriage and two daughters, ages 16 and nine, with his second wife. Tim has worked as a quality control technician at a soft drink plant for 34 years. He wants to live to be 88, so he can walk his youngest daughter down the aisle. Tim's micros include playing in a band and daily Bible reading. "I read the Bible every day at least half an hour to meditate."

## — Gautam —

Gautam is 66, married with two adult sons, and works full time as a government accountant. He was born in India but has been in the US for about 35 years. A vegetarian, he walks every day for about 15 to 20 minutes and is up at 5:30 a.m. He doesn't eat much sugar or drink alcohol.

Gautam's micromotivators are yoga and tea, and a growing sense of spirituality. He sees healthy behavior as a prerequisite for inner happiness. The two combine to give him a perspective that supports his healthy lifestyle. About three days a week, he does about 15 minutes of yoga with his wife, followed by tea, before going to work. "I like yoga. It's difficult to continuously do that, but, once you do it, you feel better. I like the feeling it gives."

### Connecting the Dots

Do you use any micromotivators? You have seen what I do to support my healthy lifestyle and the tactics of some of the men. Are there any special things you do, any little quirks or rituals that keep you on the pathway of healthy living—maybe some tactics that you've tried but never permanently adopted? If so, congratulations! Keep up the good work and stay focused on developing more. You can never have too many micros, and be sure to share them with your brothers still climbing the mountain of health. They could use a hand. If you have not yet found your micromotivators, let's look at ways you can develop your own portfolio and use them to accelerate your journey to healthy behavior.

## The Ground Rules

The ground rules for developing and utilizing micromotivators are that there are no ground rules. Micromotivators are what you say they are. No matter how basic, how crazy, or how small, you decide. The only criteria are that they work for you and help you get to the social or behavioral practice you've determined you want or need to achieve.

Your process for identifying micros can take many forms. In view of the goal of living healthy one day at a time, as I do, you can contemplate ways in which you might add some micros throughout the course of your day. Another approach that I describe below is to consider your strengths or weaknesses, leveraging your strengths to address the weaknesses through some nuanced applications.

Focusing on the factors that give you pleasure and injecting them into what otherwise might be tedious situations (i.e., a coffee and paper at 4 a.m.) is yet another way to build your micro inventory. Keep an open mind. Consider all options and be creative.

## Where to Start

Start by considering the behavioral gaps you identified back in the Chapter 4 exercises. This is a great place to begin. If there is any area in which you need support, it's in those areas that you've identified as a behavioral gap. Diet and exercise are classic targets, but don't stop there.

Instead, reflect back on your motivational planning process and the goals you've established. How's your progress? Could you use some help? Are there components in your playbook that need a boost? Do you need something to kick-start one or more of your key methods? Take a fresh look at your blueprint for healthy living.

Are you following the plan? If not, try using micromotivators to repair this breach of your personal contract with yourself.

## Ask Yourself Some Questions

Once you've zeroed-in on some areas that require a boost, conduct an inventory of strengths and weaknesses, assets, and liabilities to generate ideas for micropractices. Here are a couple of sample question sets to demonstrate the technique. They'll get your creative juices flowing and produce some ideas for your own micros.

What are the most significant barriers to the behavior I want to adopt? How can I turn this around?

- Sample answer: Getting up early to work out.
- Sample microstrategy builder:
    - If I'm up early to work out, is there anything else that I could accomplish?
    - How could some new morning rituals influence the balance of my day?
    - What would it take to make me feel good about getting up early?
- Sample microleverage: I didn't realize how beneficial it could be to get up early.

Besides consistently getting a great workout, I'm able to accomplish things that make my day and life much better. I've made a completely new set of friends at the gym (we call ourselves the Early Bird Club), gotten a jump-start on my email, and can occasionally call my daughter in Europe all before 10 a.m. As tough as it was to adopt to my new schedule, now I'm all in!

What resources can I bring to bear on the achievement of my goals that I haven't utilized?

- Sample answer: My wife has said she'd like to walk every night after dinner.

- Sample microstrategy builder:
  - My wife and I now walk together every night and track our mileage.
  - We have a discussion topic or agenda for each night's walk.
  - We've set up a practice of alternating between my wife and me for the responsibility of selecting the discussion topic.

- Sample microleverage:
  - I accomplished expanding my fitness regimen and I've simultaneously enhanced my social agenda by strengthening my relationship with my wife.

  - It's been great fun researching and preparing the discussion topics, and we're walking further and further every day!

One final approach in stimulating thought is to consider the various categories and topics that can serve as micromotivators. Here are some that I use:

### Functional Micros
- Well-being or spiritual activities
- Intellectual or interest-related activities
- Planning or analytical actions

### Social Micros
- Family
- Engagement with individuals in social relationships
- Social functions
- Fun-producing activities

- Travel/vacation Plans
- Upcoming milestone events/accomplishments

**Business Micros**
- Important meetings
- Presentations
- Evaluations
- Business milestones

**Personal Growth Micros**
- Opportunities to learn and grow intellectually
- Classes, seminars, or workshops
- Arts and entertainment-related opportunities

In this chapter, I suggested that your gap analysis from Chapter 4 would be a good place to start in your application of micromotivators. The following exercise builds on three of the five factors that comprised the Healthy Lifestyle Questionnaire. Do you have BMI of 18.5-24? Do you always or most of the time exercise at least 20 minutes, and do you regularly eat fruits and vegetables? The other two standards, do you wear a seat belt and do you smoke, fall within our guidelines and are worthy of consideration if they are indeed a problem for you, but for now I'll focus on these three, inasmuch as they represent the most significant gaps among a wide range of men.

Micromotivators are present in all facets of your life. Relative to your major social and behavioral goals in life, they are small and perhaps somewhat innocuous. They provide the daily dose of support you need on any given day, so they're often short-term in nature. They may be repetitive but still provide you with inspiration, joy, and fulfillment on an ongoing basis. They're likely right in front of you, so recognize them for the value they represent. The common denominator is that they all, in some way, shape, or form, support or contribute to the motivation of your healthy behavior. Remember, the little things can make a big difference!

When I think about micromotivators, I think about them as having the potential for what I call "adjacent relationships." That is, the micromotivators exist and have utility in influencing the task at hand because they can exist in some adjacent space. My morning coffee, the enjoyment of the solitude that enables me to think strategically about my day ahead, and my ability to get a jump on the morning news are all activities adjacent to the core purpose of getting up to go to the gym. These factors have a positive impact on my day before I hit the office—something that makes me feel good and inspires me to get up. The mental simulation that transpires in the adjacent space, and my ability to produce a benefit from what otherwise is dead space, is what amazingly flips what might normally be a tedious task into an enjoyable moment and one that contributes to the long-term sustainability of the goal. Behold the power of the micro!

## Chapter 9 Exercises

Chapter 9 is about finding the silver lining buried deep within the drudgery of healthy behavior, by finding leverage in what appears to be the mundane. Can you take lemons and make lemonade from what might otherwise be the monotony of daily life? That's the essence of micromotivation: digging deeply and with a creative mindset, matching your most at-risk behaviors with small, but significant, interventions that are transformative.

The strategy presented in Chapter 9 is, at worst, a maneuver to mitigate the most unappealing elements of your lifestyle architecture and, at best, a pathway to completely overturn any negativity and create a positive experience to which you look forward. What differentiates the micromotivator strategy is its broader, coupling nature with other factors in your life. Micromotivators are free to pull inspiration from other aspects of your life beyond the immediate circle of diet and exercise. As my examples have shown, they can extend into business, social, or other dimensions of your world, creating a productive and enjoyable alignment from what may seem tedious on the surface, like waking up at 4 a.m.

What's the methodology to do this? How can you stimulate the creative thinking to uncover these opportunities? Based on what I've learned from the men I studied, your simple step for Chapter 9 is to answer the following questions, which will set you on a path to find the motivations you need. The good news is that most of the infrastructure, the background you'll need, is already available if you completed the previous exercises. Discovering the microstrategies that can leverage your strengths and gaps is now the task at hand. Here you go.

---

### STEP 1: ID YOUR TARGETS

---

1. Where could you use a boost from a micromotivator?

2. What are the most pressing needs and the specific nature and logistics behind these needs?

3. Can you identify five targets where micros might help?

---

### STEP 2: ID MICROINTERVENTIONS

---

With a thorough understanding of your targeted areas, you can now zero-in on potential microinterventions. The interventions are often tangential to the functional target. These are the adjacent relationships discussed in the chapter. So, as you consider the possibilities, think broadly. Ask yourself questions like:

1. What else do I <u>need to accomplish</u> (that day, that week, or that month)?

2. What <u>general needs</u> do I have during or adjacent to the targeted behavior?

3. What time is available <u>adjacent</u> to the targeted behavior?

4. What time or productivity opportunities are available <u>during</u> the targeted behavior?

5. What installments can I make towards my needs, adjacent to or during the targeted behavior?

6. Is there anything that could make the unappealing behavior more appealing?

7. How will this healthy behavior make me feel today and prepare me for the day ahead?

Questions like these and others that you can certainly develop, will begin to open your eyes to a number of ideas for activities that you can wrap around your targeted vulnerabilities and lay the foundation for incorporating other (micro) actions along with the healthy behavior.

---

## STEP 3: GROW YOUR MICROS

---

Establishing you first few micros is a big deal. Congratulations! Consistent with prior strategies, track their contribution to your lifestyle. Measure their impact to determine if they are having the intended effect of mitigating the unappealing behavior, or more. Gauge their overall effectiveness, tweak as necessary, and, if not effective after a fair test period, stop the intervention. However, what's important is constantly growing your portfolio of micros. As you perfect the use of micros and witness their effectiveness, the key is to troll constantly the behavioral waters for new ones. Even ones that serve you well may be ripe for replacement if other, more effective and attractive ones come along.

Are there additional areas where micros might apply?

1. Is there a twist in an existing micro that could make life easier in a particular situation?

2. Have you shared your microstrategy with anyone? Do they use micros in any form?

# 10

# Diversify

BUSINESSES WANT A DIVERSE customer base, investors want diversity in their portfolios, and consumers demand a diverse selection of products and services: think cable TV. In a word, diversity is good. It represents choice, the ability to customize our lives, and makes the most of what the world has to offer. Diversity is a hedge against the downside and gives us the impetus to try things we might not otherwise consider.

So, too, is the case with motivation and healthy behavior. My research shows that healthy men derive their motivation from a diverse set of factors and employ a wide range of strategies to live healthily. The scope of options represented within the categories I've cited demonstrates that men seeking to live healthily can do so in any number of ways: a proverbial menu of lifestyle options. And, as you've seen in the men's stories, many of them leverage their social-motivational assets in concert with behavior, exhibiting MCBA. Bob's delight in swimming with his grandchildren is but one of the many examples.

Diversity is as fundamental to motivation and behavior as it is to business and investing. It ties back to the design of your motivational goals, implementation strategies, and partnerships. It supports sustainability and even touches on the micromotivations. A deeper look into diversity strengthens your awareness and helps you incorporate this principle into your thinking across all 10 Steps to healthy behavior.

My purpose is simple. By emphasizing the value of diversity in your planning and execution, I believe that you'll produce a more robust, interesting, and sustainable lifestyle, and be prepared for the pitfalls, to beat back the challenges, and to seize the opportunities to grow. Opening your mind to the widest set of social and behavioral prospects will enable you to exceed the 11-year benchmark of consistent behavior seen in the men I studied.

Whether it's walking up and down the stairs several times a day, doing yard-work, walking on your lunch hour, hitting the gym, walking the dog, playing with the grandchildren, or leveraging the anticipation of your next trip to finish your run, it's about being active and maintaining the motivation to stay active. Remember, the only rule is that there are no rules.

Let's start the conversation with a look back at what the healthy men told me. Examining the data that portrays motivational factors, priorities, benefits, and tactics, with an eye on diversity, sheds a new light on the findings and drives home the point that motivation and the resulting behavior choices that lead to good health are all around you.

## Motivation

Men find motivation in many places. The survey findings demonstrate this diversity. In the study, the men ranked 21 motivating factors. They considered 12 somewhat or most motivating' while nine was less motivating. Some of the less motivating still received respectable ratings at over 35%. The high rankings represent the reliance men place on such a broad list of inspiration.

Factors considered most motivating, rated from 66% to 76%, demonstrated the influence they wield. They range from fear over loss of mental ability at 66% to fear over loss of physical ability receiving the top ranking at 76%. The span of responses represents the variety of underlying values, lifestyles, and personal circumstances on the men's minds. While the highest-rated sources of motivation will likely ring true with a large number of men, the fact that the ratings are both highly ranked and tightly grouped reinforce the multiplicity of influence.

Somewhat motivating factors rated between 45% and 56%. Responses ranged from experienced illness or injury at 45%, to concern about relationship with, spouse or significant other at 56%. In between are factors such as ability to enjoy a hobby and concern over my appearance or weight.

Even some of the more significant among the less motivating factors category received respectable ratings such as spouse's recommendation at 40% and enjoy my grandchildren at 37%. This offers further evidence of the depth of diversity.

## Priorities

Priorities play a major role in providing motivation. The findings include measures of eight life's priorities grouped in three categories including high priority, somewhat of a priority, and much lower priority. While the eight factors that men rate is less than the 19 under motivation, the results are consistent in that they reflect diversity in content and a respectable degree of impact. The sole high priority rating, time with wife/significant other tops out at 73%, followed with a mix of three factors listed as somewhat of a priority; travel, time with children, and hobbies. Much lower priorities are equally diverse, yet still receive respectable ratings, mostly in the 30th percentile. In sum, the survey produced a smorgasbord of priorities that fuel motivation.

## Benefits

Men's ratings on the benefits of living healthy are further testimony in the case for diversity. They rated and clustered the 15 points into four categories: highest value, high value, some value, and lowest value. The items reconcile with the motivations and priorities and offer some unique insights that further define the message of diversity.

Among the 15, the lowest value, ability to serve my church, ranked at 29%, while the highest-rated point is absence of debilitating illness/sickness at 96%. This wide span and the variance of factors within the range support the case that men derive a variety of perceived benefits, which fuels their behavior. Factors within this range include ability to maintain an active sex life, ability to travel, and ability to maintain my independence. The weight given to each factor shows the significance of the benefits on men's behavior. Seven benefits scored between 74% and 96%, and 5 received ratings between 52% and 69%, all great scores.

## Tactics

With diversity well-established in men's motivations, priorities, and perceived benefits, I now turn to the tactics used to channel behavior. Here again, the men's answers scream diversity. Among the 12 factors rated, six ranked above 40%, and all exhibited a variety of applications to both diet and exercise/activity. I also found continued strong showings and a heavy reliance on multiple items in both diet and exercise. For example, among the highest-rated items include meal planning, 68%; exercise on the same schedule; 62%, and building exercise into vacations, 61%. Lower rated, but still significant, were: using exercise or my hobby as time to reflect on personal or work-related issues, 52%; maintaining a contingency plan, 43%; and engaging in exercise or a hobby with a spouse/family or friend, 44%.

The findings are clear. Whether it's the motivating factors, men's priorities, perceived benefits, or the tactics that guide behaviors, the menu of inspiration and resulting behavior is expansive. So, as you contemplate which factors may hold the greatest potential to drive healthy behavior in your life, and which best match your circumstances, think broadly, don't limit your considerations. Just pretend you have the cable TV remote in your hand and hundreds of options from which to choose. Trust me, you'll find your motivational networks and the behavior channels that match your tastes.

## My Dad

As I write this chapter, our family is planning my father's 90th birthday. He's amazing. He drives, lives independently with a woman he met maybe 20 years ago (my mother and he divorced probably 35-40 years ago), goes dancing every Friday night, and hits a local McDonald's three days a week, where a group of seniors transform the restaurant into a senior center every morning, bingo included. An attorney by trade, he practiced law well into his 80s and still gives advice to many inquiring seniors at McDonald's. Yes, he's quite the active guy.

Now, besides the gratitude, I feel for the transmission of his genes and, more so, for his fatherly guidance and love over the years. As I prepared his biography for the birthday party, I realized that my dad represents a case study in motivational diversity. Over the years his interests—his priorities and motivations—have changed and evolved, providing him with a continual wellspring of inspiration that's produced his active lifestyle. In some cases, these motivations drove physical behaviors, but, overall, they demonstrate how a man can find the drive for an active lifestyle in a variety of sources.

While some of Dad's diversification is the result of a normal evolution of life and the maturing of his family (and consequently a topic for a later chapter in this book, Adjust with Age), I think the body of his life's work more significantly exemplifies diversity. The assorted directions of his interests over time may come from his children but have evolved well beyond them. Rather, I would argue that Dad's life represents a penchant for trying new things and enjoying the excitement he derives from those experiences. I still see it today, in the stories he tells about his new friends at McDonald's. Accordingly, I have included it here.

## The Kids

Let's start with my siblings and me. I'm the oldest of five. There are three sisters (two of whom are twins), my brother, and me. As I look back, our ages, interests, and genders represent one entry in Dad's diversified portfolio that, from all accounts, continues to create a lot of inspiration for him. My route was traditional for a child growing up in the 60s and 70s: Little League baseball, school-related sports, activities (I was a drummer), and the like. The point is, Dad was there, umpiring the Little League games, attending the school show to hear my drum solo, and ultimately returning letters I would write to him from college, correcting my spelling and punctuation errors. More college stories ahead, but Dad's plunge into my childhood certainly indicates a man motivated by engaging with his children.

For the twins, it was a shift to softball and, for one of them, basketball. One summer, he even started an ad hoc softball team with my sisters and a bunch of girls at the local field, when we were away on vacation. For my third sister, it was field hockey, and then soccer for my brother—even more diversity.

Somewhere in this mix, when I was in high school in the late 60s, early 70s, and before my parents had divorced, Dad got the bug to start a softball team at our church. In this case, his energy literally turned into a physical dimension, as he purchased t-shirts, contacted other Catholic parishes, and recruited players (including a couple of my teenage buddies and me) for the team. Dad pitched and was our leader. We played on Sundays, had a great time, and created many memories, yet another activity.

Back to soccer: My brother's interest in soccer prompted Dad's immersion into the sport and its international dimensions. Besides learning all about this sport, which was certainly new to a kid who grew up on baseball and football, soccer struck a chord with Dad through his Croatian heritage. I can remember back when my brother was a soccer player in high school and college, and Dad was diving headfirst into the Olympics, World Cup, and other international soccer competition, where he closely followed the teams from his native Split, Croatia, in what was then Yugoslavia. It carried him to a completely new dimension in his life, created strong bonds with my brother, and even prompted travel that included a trip to the Summer Olympics in Los Angeles and other junkets. Talk about keeping the fires burning in your belly. Soccer was a big factor for a stretch.

## The Grandchildren

Dad's interests advanced to another new level as grandchildren came onto the scene. Two stories exemplify his commitment to his grand-children and the inspiration they provided.

He was a staple during the childhood sports careers of my two sons, Anthony and Stephen. One of my fondest memories is the season when my older son, Anthony, my dad, and I would film Steve's midget football games and get them aired on the local cable access channel. Our three-man crew included Dad as cameraman, Anthony as executive producer, and me as the on-field reporter who would interview the coach and star players before and after the game. Yes, I would literally put on a suit (or just keep the suit on from work for a Friday night game), stand there with a fake microphone (the real mike was on the video camera), and play reporter by interviewing 12-year-olds after the game. It is amazing what we do for our kids!

The kids and the parents loved watching their sons, (girls did not play competitive football in those days), on the local cable channel, and we all thought it was a hoot. Most importantly, we bonded and Dad loved the experience. It was the ultimate multidimensional motivational activity. Dad was with his son and grandsons, enjoying the game and living his hobby and secret dream as a cameraman. He thought life couldn't get much better. Give this a try!

As cool and inspiring as it was for Dad to interact with his grandsons, it was the diversity of his granddaughters that took him to yet another dimension of being a grandfather. My sister Terry has two daughters, both of whom were All-American softball players at major college programs: Oklahoma and Florida. As my nieces progressed through their collegiate careers, Dad was there. Through several trips to their games, he got to know the coaches and players. He followed them on television and over the internet (often asking me to look up recent games on the internet and print out hard-copy stories of their games). However, by far, the most exciting times occurred when my nieces were in the Softball World Series. Coming from top sports programs at their universities, they were fortunate to have the experience. I can recall watching them on ESPN, and, of course, seeing Dad in the stands all clad in his team's swag, cheering them on. By then, his film interests had moved to still photography, so he'd come back from the trips with tons of pictures with the girls, coaches, and, of course, my sister and his granddaughters. This was very cool, and, for him, just another inspiring reason to stay active and healthy.

**Dancing**

So, what does Dad do to stay limber? What was his go-to strategy over the years, particularly once his softball days were over? The answer is dancing. Yes, Dad is a dancer. Call it jitterbug or swing, today at 90, he remains a product of the big band era. His ritual is a light dinner and dancing every Friday night with his girl (in her 90s as well), and every New Year's Eve. It's something to which he looks forward. It gives him photographs to show at McDonald's and stories to share. Yes, stories about the other couples, their nuances, and the funny things that happen.

## Dad's Summary

It is certainly a wonderful thing to be able to look back on your parent's life and be able to cite so many wonderful memories. On that count, I plead guilty. However, my point in telling you about my dad is very purposeful and relevant to our conversation about healthy behavior. Dad was not, and is not, a gym-goer or exercise fanatic. He never followed any special diet. He's gone through periods where his weight has fluctuated, although he was never a heavy guy. He just watches what he eats and keeps things in moderation.

Dad has had some heart issues, which he manages well, and he had an encounter with prostate cancer, which has also been dormant for some time. He is just a very active man who has been able to make it to 90 and sustain his active lifestyle. At the heart of his story is a diversity of motivation that includes his children and grandchildren; his hobbies of film, photography, and travel; and his interest in his Croatian ancestry. If there is anything you can take from Dad's life so far, (who knows what's next!), it's his willingness to embrace diversity and change.

## Diversity Mapping Tips:

### Level-Set

Measure your current level of diversity in your lifestyle architecture. Are all your motivational and behavioral eggs in just a few baskets? Would new, additional inspiration help? Consistent with the message in Chapter 4, you need to assess where you are now when it comes to your behavior. Such is also the case when considering your degree of diversity found in your motivations and behaviors.

### Look Back to Plan Ahead

Where can you look for inspiration? We've seen all the examples from our men, so try this. Think about what made you happy as a kid, teenager, or young adult. Are there activities or interests that you can pull out of mothballs now that you have the time? Did you play an instrument? Did you paint or draw? Were you a reader? Did you feel rewarded through volunteer work? Have you considered a social cause in which to become involved? Would you like to get closer to distant family members with whom you might have lost touch? The list continues.

### Research New Things

Finally, there are many new opportunities to travel, volunteer, and engage in activities like never before. Many of these opportunities are for individuals or you can participate with a spouse or partner, children, or even grandchildren. The internet offers an immediate connection to whole host of options, if you're inclined. Personally, I'm working on some sports fan-oriented road trips with my boys.

Build your own diversity map in the exercise that follows. It will lead you to the destination of a lifetime!

# Chapter 10 Exercises

Chapter 10 is about building a diverse portfolio of social motivators, continually looking for new endeavors that can keep your interests fresh and your inspiration for healthy living strong. You've seen the examples offered by my dad, and I've just ended the chapter with a few tips to guide you in your personal diversity mapping. Picking up on the three tips, answer the following questions. They'll provide the simple steps you need to begin the process of expanding your inventory of go-to motivators, reinforce your commitment to healthy behavior, and maybe even add a little more fun in your life. Try this out.

### Level-Set Questions: Be a Dreamer

1.  Can you identify five new social activities that will give you something to look forward to every day?

2. Maybe something that you've always wanted to do, but just never tried?

3. Perhaps an activity that a friend or colleague has been urging you to take up with them?

4. A spin-off of something you enjoy now?

## Looking Back to Plan Ahead: Be a Historian

1. Can you list at least three activities, hobbies, or relationships that were particularly rewarding in your childhood or earlier in your life?

2. Does the thought of re-engaging in these activities or relationships create a spark of excitement?

3. What would it take to rekindle these activities?

## Research a Few New Things: Be an Explorer

1. Have you ever done any research to stimulate your thinking on new social motivators?

2. Have you discussed your desire to expand your social motivators with your spouse, partner, family, or friends?

3. Have you attended any meetings, lectures, or read up on potential social opportunities as a way to identify new endeavors?

# 11

# Be Optimistic

OPTIMISM INFLUENCES HEALTHY BEHAVIOR. The psychology literature documents the correlation between optimism and healthy behavior. The healthy men I spoke to confirmed it. Of the men I polled, 60% considered themselves optimistic and 75% of these same men indicated that optimism is an important factor for maintaining a healthy lifestyle. All the 10 men I interviewed in one of my focus groups considered themselves optimistic and agreed that optimism contributed to their ability to sustain a healthy lifestyle. Is this a coincidence?

The difference a positive attitude makes is something I've witnessed throughout my entire life. As a kid playing sports, I remember the coaches preaching the importance of a positive attitude, and observing some of the boys hanging tough when we were losing while others seemed to melt down. The phrase "keep your head up" bellowed from the coaches still rings in my head after all these years. In fact, when my boys were growing up, I frequently witnessed how they excelled in their performance when they displayed a positive attitude toward the challenge, whether it was sports, homework, or other school activities.

As a sports fan, I often hear sports talk radio callers rambling on about the attitude of professional athletes and its impact on their performance. In business, assessing the attitude of job applicants and their level of enthusiasm is a standard operating practice.

Yes, attitude, and specifically optimism, is an integral part of a healthy lifestyle and, therefore, warrants inclusion in our conversation. But, there's more. One can link optimism with longer life. Optimism is important in countless other ways that improve your personal and social life and enhance your psychological well-being. Behavioral scientists indicate that optimism can help blunt loneliness (Rius-Ottenheim, Kromhout, Mast, Zitman, Geleijnse, & Giltay, 2011), support better relationships, promote conflict resolution, extend relationships, and generate coping strategies (Carver, Sheier & Segerstom, 2010). Wow! Talk about a value-added proposition.

Further, the research contains particularly good news for 50+ men. Scientists indicate that, as you age, you are very much in control of our own emotional health, unlike the inevitable decline experienced in other areas of health. Aging, per se, does not generally negatively affect a person's emotional health. In fact, research suggests that we experience more positive and less negative emotions as we get older, (partially because we proactively select only the most emotionally rewarding social relationships.) Cognitive style and other individual differences are much more important in determining your emotional health (Dionigi, 2015). The bottom line is that your attitude counts, and in a very big way.

Now let's be clear, these same scientists tell us that if you're not naturally an optimist becoming one is hard work. However, it's not impossible and there are clinical interventions as well as do-it-yourself practical tips that you can follow to help adopt and maintain an optimistic attitude.

## Personal Optimism vs. External Pessimism

Optimism is the overall view that the world is a great place and that things will turn out okay. According to preeminent positive psychologist Dr. Martin Seligman, optimists:

Believe that defeat is just a temporary setback, that its causes are confined to just one case—defeat is not their fault. Not only do optimists generally believe that things will ultimately turn out for the best, but when bad things do happen, they don't fault themselves, but external, often uncontrollable, yet temporary events, and most importantly, they don't dwell on it.

Most people are generally optimistic about things that have turned out well for them in the past, or about things that have good associations for them. People can also be optimistic about their internal lives and still pessimistic about external world events (Seligman, 2006).

To me, this distinction is extremely significant and relates directly to our conversation about the health and behavior of men 50+. Yes, there are many reasons to be pessimistic about the world today, a point I will elaborate on shortly. However, in my experience, the strongest source of motivation and optimism—and the one source with the ability to overcome these world-based depressing messages— is our families and our life's priorities. While pollsters may measure society's overall optimism or pessimism based on worldviews, there is no reason why you can't narrow your focus to more immediate factors: those that you can control and those that have meaning that is more direct to your life.

## Blind Optimism

A short caveat is appropriate to address the concept of extreme blind optimism and rule this out of the conversation. No one is suggesting that optimism should be based on anything but reality. What behaviorists call blind optimism is not necessarily a productive or preferred trait. Becoming more optimistic does not mean blinding yourself to the dangers of the world. Dr. Seligman advises that "there are times and places where we need our pessimism." Seligman's general rule of thumb for when not to use optimism is, "If the cost of failure is high, optimism is the wrong strategy." (Seligman, 2006). At times throughout our lives, we find ourselves in high stakes situations where a little worrying and being prepared for possible negative outcomes in the future can be very important. This is a good point to keep in mind as we go forward.

## A Strong Association with Positive Health Outcomes

A wealth of research has found that optimism is strongly associated with a wide variety of positive health outcomes, such as slower disease progression, increased immune functioning, lower rates of cardiovascular disease, and increased survival rates in certain types of cancer. The research also shows that at least one important factor in choosing to engage in health-conscious behaviors is optimism (Rassmussen, Scheier, & Greenhouse, 2009).

Various studies report that optimism is positively linked with eating more fresh fruits and vegetables (Kelloniemi, Ek, & Laitinen, 2005), non-smoking, and less alcohol intake in older individuals (Steptoe, Wright, Kunz-Ebrecht, & Iliffe, 2006). Giltay, et al. (2007) also found that participants who showed high levels of optimism were significantly more likely to be more physically active, avoid smoking, drink less alcohol, and eat healthier. In sum, optimistic people tend to be healthier because they tend to eat and act healthier. This relationship also works in the other direction. Someone who is less optimistic could engage in less healthy behaviors, which could lead to negative health outcomes. These undesirable results could lower their optimism even more, since it makes sense that developing health issues could very well take a toll on your disposition. Are you convinced?

## Staying in Rhythm

Earlier in the book, I spoke about the value of rhythm in your lifestyle architecture and the ability to stay in rhythm or get back in rhythm when life's road bumps throw you off. I also shared the personal experiences that challenged me as a young man—the death of my unborn son, two divorces, and some very public professional battles—and described how exercise and healthy behavior kept me going. In truth, optimism contributed greatly to my ability to get through these times and sustain my rhythm. Despite the pattern of some profoundly negative circumstances, which could have pulled me backwards, a healthy dose of optimism was a key ingredient in creating a cycle of behavior that ultimately became a self-perpetuating lifeline that carried me through some very dark days.

What is the source of my optimism? It is no secret: my life's priorities are my source of optimism. Depending on the point in time, a future with the kids, the opportunity to have a successful career (and ability to provide for the kids), and finding the love of my life—just to name a few factors—fueled my optimistic fires.

So, if the psychology isn't enough to convince you that optimism has health benefits and prompt you to approach life differently, then consider this. In my journey through life, and specifically through my 20s into my 40s, I came upon many intersections. Those intersections represented very personal decision points. I could wallow in the misfortune and very justifiable pessimism that had confronted me or, I could consider the opportunities that the future held and the potential to advance my personal goals despite the circumstances I faced. A mental inventory of those possibilities made it a no-brainer. Optimism was my preferred path. So far, almost 20 years later, I'd say it was the right choice.

My story illustrates what many men regularly encounter in their lives: choices. While the circumstances leading to your choices are no doubt different, what we have in common is the ability to choose optimism. While you may be in a position where pessimism, or even depression, may seem like a very rational and fact-based choice, the experts remind us that it is not.

As you proceed through life, particularly into your later years, you can be optimistic and derive the health benefits that optimism brings or lean elsewhere. Personally, I haven't found the down side to optimism. I don't think it exists. Nevertheless, many of our 50+ brothers won't drink the Kool Aid of optimism. Yes, many have individual stories that would certainly seem to warrant anything but optimism. Unemployment, loss of a spouse or partner and other life challenges can breed depression and discouragement. The growth of behavioral health as a diagnosis certainly demonstrates the enormity of the challenge to be optimistic (Twenge, 2015). Still, my point is simply to make you aware of the upside and the tremendous impact that optimism can have on your health.

## Perspective from Health-Conscious Men

I asked 10 men if they considered themselves optimistic and if their optimism made a positive contribution to their lifestyle. All 10 said yes to both while also exhibiting the internal-external based optimism-pessimism phenomenon. The diversity of viewpoints demonstrates how different roads can lead to the same destination and, no matter what your situation, you can tailor your course.

— **Tom** —

Tom, a 78-year-old tour guide, expresses confidence about his optimistic approach to life:

> I understand that there's two sides to almost every issue.
> And, I like to think that either I can influence the outcome,
> and it would be a positive outcome if I'm influencing it.
> And so, I think that's kind of optimistic.

He continues:

> And, I think—and many, many things work out well. Sometimes they don't. That's just the way life is. But I like to feel that—I don't feel that the world is against me or that the sky is going to fall tomorrow. I like to feel that whatever the situation is, I'm going to be able to handle it, and I'm going to make it work out well is basically, my philosophy on life.

## — Rod —

Rod, the 66-year-old retired corporate executive who now works as a self-employed carpenter, describes himself as a glass-half-full guy. "There's a lot of negative things out in this world that we have to be aware of or recognize—but there's more good out there, and I'm pretty much optimistic in that sense."

As for the impact on his behavior, Rod said, "I never sat down and thought of that, but in some sense it must. You know, it's got to influence it (healthy behavior) in some way or another."

## — Tim —

You remember Tim, the 52-year-old quality control technician who works for a soft-drink company. The seeds of his optimism stem from a childhood experience that carries through to today:

> I always know somebody's got it worse. I always tell my kids that. When you think you have it bad, there's somebody out there—I had a bad hip when I was a kid and I was in Shriners Hospital when I was, I guess, about 10 years old. I remember being all depressed. Why do I got to go to the hospital? Because I was born with a defective hip, and I went and looked around and I was like… cursing God the whole way. And I got there, and it was like, "Thank you, God." There were kids there with no

legs, severely deformed. And, I'm like, all I got is a bad hip? And people don't even know now.

And, when it comes to the impact of optimism on his behavior, Tim has a lot to say:

> I just think happy people live longer. And, if you're optimistic, you're happy. And, I know I'll live longer because of it. I don't worry about things I can't control. It drives my wife nuts sometimes. But, if I can't change it, I'm not going to worry about it.

## — Harris —

Harris is a 53-year-old insurance broker. He characterizes himself as internally optimistic:

> Sometimes I get mad about things I see on the news, and that may make me look negative. But, I think, ultimately, I want everything to be happy and be good, you know. I think it's important to be as optimistic as you can be in here (pointing to his head). I know inside I'm optimistic. And, it probably is what keeps me from, at least so far, not getting anything major.

## — Robert —

Robert is a 62-year-old human resources executive. "I consider myself extremely optimistic—there's nothing that can't be overcome or can't be done. I mean no matter what the issue is."

Robert's take on the role of optimism in supporting healthy behavior is:

> I think it definitely does, because I think if I didn't have a positive outlook about things, it would be easy to get depressed. It would be easy to overeat. It would be easy

to smoke and drink. You know, be merry and drink and have fun in the excess because it's, you know, nothing beyond this very moment. So, I think my outlook definitely shaped—has shaped—my thrust toward healthy living, which, to me, it's just a foundation.

## — Kevin —

Kevin is a 53-year-old musician and bandleader who married later in life and has three children, ages eight through 12. He's a classic example of the individual who is pessimistic about the world but optimistic about his personal and internal life. Kevin is involved in local politics where he lives and immediately responds to my question about optimism with a firm statement, "I'm more pessimistic than optimistic."

However, when I dig deeper and suggest that he leave politics out of the equation and focus on his personal life and his healthy behavior, his response is quite different:

"I think I'm optimistic," he says and, after more conversation, reveals a much more deep-rooted optimistic perspective. "I think there is always hope for people that are out of shape and want to try to get in shape and live a healthy lifestyle. There is—there's always hope in people. They can do it."

## Other Perspectives on Optimism and Pessimism

Despite all the documented benefits of optimism, experts indicate that most people say they are pessimistic. One perspective is that, like many things, such either/or choices don't reflect the nuances of real life. Optimism and pessimism can co-exist and vary, depending on circumstances. By example, they suggest that you may have an optimistic outlook on life but feel quite pessimistic about your job. They recommend that you think of optimism as a sliding scale, one end being extremely optimistic and the other being very low on optimism, with all of us fitting somewhere along this scale (Seligman, 2006).

Others argue that if we just look at contemporary society from a historical perspective, there are many reasons for optimism, and that short-term obsessions largely influence pessimism in the US, which are products of the 24-hour news cycle. A 2014 article by Morgan Housel published in *USA Today* (Fool, 2014) listed 50 reasons to be optimistic based on advances in medicine, technology, and science that have vastly improved our quality of life. The reasons cited ranged from the fact that Americans are living longer and retiring at an average age of 62; to the number of homes, which today have electricity and refrigerators; to the huge reductions in the number of traffic fatalities.

While all true, historic references don't shape contemporary public opinion and perceptions of well-being. Surely, the media's need for ratings and content has combined to produce an obsession with a pessimistic view of the world. "If it bleeds, it leads," is a well-worn but still very much applicable characterization of our world today. On the other hand, some of the horrific tragedies that have occurred in the US over the past several years and the growth of terrorism may test even the most optimistic person's convictions.

## Can You Learn Optimism?

So, let's assume you've made the commitment to healthy living and you want to do everything possible to increase your chances for sustaining this behavior and living a long, healthy life. You're convinced that there's merit to the research that links optimism with positive health outcomes, and you understand that there is a big difference between your internal optimism and more pessimistic worldviews. Still, you aren't quite the optimistic type. Can you learn optimism? The short answer is yes, but, as I noted, it's not a walk in the park. Let's examine a high-level look at the process.

For starters, let's look at the age-old question of nature vs. nurture and see how much your parents control the situation. A 1993 (Schulman, Keith & Seligman, 1993) study of identical twins showed that 25% inherited both optimism and pessimism, thus leaving room for other influences. Accordingly, researchers found that environmental factors, including family environment, strongly influence both optimism and pessimism (Bates, 2015). So, while somewhat influenced by genetics and your childhood, the experts suggest that yes, you can learn optimism.

In his book, *The Undefeated Mind*, Dr. Alex Lickerman cites explanatory flexibility as one approach to learning to be more optimistic. Explanatory flexibility is a willingness to reformulate how you think about the causes of negative events and work towards a realistic, but optimistic, self-explanatory style that balances the way you evaluate the causes of negative life events without surrendering your sense of power and control over them. To demonstrate that changing your self-explanatory style can make a difference and help produce more optimistic thinking, Dr. Lickerman offered two great examples (Lickerman, 2012).

In one study, Lickerman trained male basketball players to attribute positive results—making a free throw—to their *ability* and negative results to their *lack of effort*. He found that it significantly improved their subsequent performance. Another study showed optimism training increased the persistence with which novice golfers attempted to improve their game. Lickerman's conclusion: How you explain the causes of your problems (like failing to make a putt) almost certainly plays an important role in determining how you respond to them, and the stories you tell yourself about why bad things happen really do affect what happens next (Lickerman, 2012).

So, besides telling yourself the right things when life doesn't go your way, what other steps can you take to be more optimistic? The internet is full of handy tips. Here's just one sample that does a good job of summarizing some of the most common tactics.

## Tips on Becoming Optimistic

Optimism doesn't mean ignoring the hard or challenging things in life, but it does mean changing how you approach them. If you've always had a pessimistic worldview, it can be difficult to re-orient your perspective, but it is possible to highlight the positive in your life with a little patience and mindfulness (Seligman, 2006).

When pessimism and negative beliefs do come up, Seligman suggests that the following four strategies can help you effectively dispute those thoughts and get your mind back on the road to optimism (Seligman, 2006).

1. Evidence: Is there really evidence for your negative belief? Or, are you just jumping to the worst-case scenario?

2. Alternatives: What are some less destructive ways to look at the situation? Remember: Focus on the *changeable,* the *specific,* and the *non-personal* causes.

3. Implications: Even if your negative belief is correct, is it really that big of a deal? Just because something bad happened, doesn't make it the end of the world.

4. Usefulness: Even if it is as bad as it seems, is it helpful to dwell on it? Just because your pessimism might be correct, doesn't make it useful.

## Motivation, Optimism & Healthy Living

Optimism is a core element in the psychology of healthy behavior. The correlation between optimism and a variety of positive health outcomes is strong, and the opportunity to adopt an optimistic view-point is there, even for those predisposed to lean more pessimistically. Those of us higher-up on the ladder of age also have access to these opportunities. As we discovered earlier in this chapter, age is not generally a factor in emotional health.

Beyond these findings from the field of psychology, my national survey bears out the value of optimism, as well as the personal interviews I conducted with healthily-behaving men.

Yes, optimism makes a difference. It is another tool in your growing tool kit of motivation. As in the other psychologically based strategies offered in this book, the actions required are largely mental, not physical—although the benefits extend when teamed with exercise and diet, and other physical dimensions of healthy behavior.

My own personal experience presents my most enduring argument for adopting an optimistic approach to life. It's an approach grounded in personal values and priorities, my most precious and meaningful treasures in life. As a young man, my boys gave me hope and inspired my optimism by way of their future and our future together. I wanted them to grow up full of optimism about life and the rewards and fulfillment it offers. Maybe it was just dumb luck, or my parents, or the circumstances that pushed me to see that the glass was half-full. Whatever, I'm glad I did and even more glad that I still do—more than ever—today. My advice to those who are hesitant to wade in the pool of optimism is simple—try it. You have nothing to lose. Optimism is not so bad. It will do wonders and may even open doors you didn't know existed.

In the exercise that follows, I'll connect you with a couple of links that can help you start on your path to optimism by helping you determine where you are on the scale of optimism and pessimism. Go for it.

## Chapter 11 Exercises

Chapter Eleven is about optimism and its place as a component of a healthy lifestyle. The sentiment found in the literature supports my research of healthily living men over 50. As you design your own lifestyle, it is important for you to assess your level of optimism. Even if you don't consider yourself an optimist, it's possible to become one. Your simple goal in this exercise is to assess your level of optimism.

Below is an inventory of tools from which you can assess your current level of optimism and create your individual optimism map. Through the exercises, you'll discover ways, in which you can find optimism in your life, develop or strengthen your level of optimism, and leverage your optimism to support healthy behavior. You'll find it interesting and thought- provoking.

For starters, to check on whether you're optimistic or pessimistic go to: http://www.seemypersonality.com/personality.asp?p=Optimism-Test#q1 where you'll be able to take a free, five-minute test to determine if you're a glass half full or glass half empty kind of person.

As a preview, below are some of the questions you'll find.

1. Do you expect the best or worst outcome?

2. Does your outlook affect your motivation?

3. Do you have trust and faith in people?

4. Do you expect the best?

5. If something can go wrong for you, will it?

6. Do good things happen to you?

If you're interested in a more extensive measure of your ability to adopt an optimistic viewpoint go to http://web.stanford.edu/class/msande271/onlinetools/LearnedOpt.html where you'll find the Learned Optimism Test developed by Stanford University, based in Dr. Martin Seligman's book *Learned Optimism*. This more extensive 48-question test takes about 15 minutes and provides an analysis based on the rules spelled out in *Learned Optimism* by Dr. Seligman.

If you're looking for some more detailed strategies try the following from http://www.wikihow.com/Be-Optimistic.

# *12*

# Adjust

CHANGE: IT'S BOTH INEVITABLE and central to your consideration of healthy behavior. Like it or not, life is not a static proposition. As you age, change enters your life through many doors. Sometimes you open the door and welcome change. Other times, change knocks down your door and is an unwelcome intruder. Either way, change is a trigger, a mechanism that prompts a reevaluation of priorities, a reassessment of your goals, and a review of the strategies, tactics, and rituals that comprise your behavior. When the underlying conditions that influenced your plans shift, you need to adjust accordingly by leveraging the opportunities and mitigating the challenges. In short, adjust.

Self-directed changes like retirement, a second career, volunteering, and travel are a result of planning and are, as such, welcomed events. Graduations, weddings, and grandchildren are emotional milestones emerging from change in the normal course of life. Imposed change, such as that brought on by physical limitations, medical conditions, or other threats on your independence can produce anxiety and threaten the lifestyle to which you've become accustomed. Yes, change is multifaceted, but the most significant dimension of change is managing it. Do you pro-actively embrace change and seize the opportunities? Does change strike fear in you? Are you ambivalent? Have you reflected on the changes you've experienced or those that lie ahead and given thought to how you might adjust your lifestyle over time?

## The Science of Change

Psychology well represents the behavioral change associated with age, offering further insights into the concept of redefining with age. Well-established models and theories make the case that men can successfully adapt to limitations, physical or cognitive, resulting from the aging process. Among the relevant theories are The Selective Optimization with Compensation model (SOC), Assimilation and Accommodation Theory, and Socio-Emotional Selectivity Theory. Collectively, these theories provide the technical and academic underpinnings borne out in the responses of the men I've studied.

It is important to note that these theories focus solely on the premise that abilities become limited and do not venture into a consideration of the power of new motivations. Coping with age is a long-studied field and it is important for you to know that researchers have developed a substantial body of literature that supports the use of strategy to sustain function. This sampling of some of the most basic theories will serve our purpose.

## The Selective Optimization with Compensation Model (SOC)

When faced with constricted resources, successful individuals tend to engage in selection, optimization, and compensation in order to adapt successfully to these limitations (Baltes, 1997). SOC suggests that, as your abilities become more limited, you can focus on the activities that are more satisfying and the skills to which you are better suited. By doing this, you can also focus more energy on these specific skills and activities and get even better at them.

You can also develop strategies to compensate for any diminished abilities. These strategies are obviously going to vary depending on the activity, but, as an example, Baltes (1997) described concert pianist, Arthur Rubinstein, in relation to how he managed to adapt his musical skills as he aged. He said that he started to play fewer pieces but practiced these pieces more often. In addition, for faster pieces that he was no longer able to do, he slowed down the previous pieces, so the relative speed was still faster.

## Assimilation and Accommodation

The basic idea behind assimilation and accommodation is that when you do encounter age-related obstacles in life, you can deal with them in two possible ways. The first, assimilation, is when you compensate for your limited abilities and even sometimes manipulate the environment to help you continue the activities you enjoy. This is very similar to the SOC. The other way, accommodation, more or less involves disengaging from those goals and focusing on achievable alternatives. This may also include devaluing those blocked goals, to reduce the emotional impact of not being able to pursue them.

The research on these mechanisms is extensive, but the bottom line is this: Ideally, you should strike a healthy balance between the two. As you age, you can't take on the world exactly the way you did when you were young, so you will have to make some concessions, and that's okay. But, that certainly doesn't mean that we have to throw in the towel on everything we want to do. Neither extreme is healthy; the goal here is to strive for a healthy balance (Brandtstadter & Greve, 1994; Brandtstadter & Rothermund, 1994; Brandtstadter, Rothermund & Schmitz, 1997; Rothermund & Brandtstadter, 2003a).

### Socio-Emotional selectivity theory

According to Carstensen (1991), peoples' social goals tend to fall into two categories: the acquisition of knowledge, and the regulation of emotion. When you're younger and you perceive that you have more time to spare, you tend to focus on the acquisition of knowledge. But, when you perceive you're shorter on time, such as in advanced age, your emotional health becomes more of a priority. In this case, you focus on strengthening and maintaining relationships with those closest and most familiar to you. Now, this is not surprising, given that in my survey, the number one priority for the men who participated was spending time with their significant others, and, notably, the older men in the survey were even more focused on spending time with their partners vs. their career and travel.

However, this can put men at a disadvantage because they tend to have smaller social networks than women do—which makes them comparatively more reliant on their partners, which in turn means they have a much harder time after losing their partner. The important take-away from this is just to keep in mind that maintaining close social relationships not only provides benefits now, but will keep you prepared for when you really need them in the future (Carstensen, L. L., Isaacowitz, D.M. & Charles, S.T., 1999).

**The Common Theme**

The common theme emerging from these theories of aging adaptation is consistent with the survey findings and the comments of the interviewees. As you age, your goals shift, as your priorities shift from intellectual and physical development to a more direct attempt to enjoy life as it is now. This may be a more difficult transition for some men than others, but the important thing to remember is that it's normal to want to focus on fewer things and fewer relationships, if those are the things that really make you happy.

**Change and Economic Opportunity**

Economically and emotionally, it's a great time for 50+ men. Studies show that in addition to providing sustainable employment for those in need, the nation's current economic state offers 50+ men new opportunities for career-oriented fulfillment and satisfaction.

The Bureau of Labor Statistics projects that the participation rate of workers 65 and older will rise to 23% in 2022. Part of this phenomenon is the incredible demographic shift that's happening globally. In today's economy, the age of one's physical peak is often divorced from the best years of productivity. Experts point to the fact that some jobs require cognitive skills considered "age-appreciating"— in other words, skills that actually improve with age. According to one research paper, these skills can be anything from technical writing to human-resources management. Some studies have shown that working (or volunteering) can be a good thing for the health of seniors (Toossi, 2013).

"Reinforcing the Non-Economic Aspects of Sustained Employment" is a study commissioned by the AARP that indicates that although current and future financial needs are a top reason that employees stay in the workforce past age 50, psychological and social fulfillment also play a role (Hewitt, 2015).

While economic factors can certainly change, the underlying demographic shifts that are producing these employment opportunities are longitudinal in nature, thus, move slowly over time. For now, it seems like there's never been a better time to be in the 50+ category and never more options to sustain the motivation to live healthily and take full advantage of this market.

## Redefining for Physical & Social Change

Physical and social changes are at the heart of redefinition. You can manage physical change in any number of ways. Several of the men I interviewed contrasted their exercise and dietary regimes as younger men to those that they've adopted with age. Many have incorporated social opportunities into these physical adaptations. A former marathoner described how he now runs 5K and 10K races with his daughter. Another gentleman, also a runner, now hikes with his grandchildren on their way to the lake where they fish. A number of the men described their migration to a diet dominated by more chicken, fish, and vegetables, in partnership with their spouse's healthy eating habits.

Social change has multiple aspects that extend from divorce to the miracle of birth. Each can be a source of motivation and each requires a management strategy. The aging of others in your life precipitates some adjustments in social relationships. As children and grandchildren age, your relationship with them evolves. You will do different things and find great satisfaction in these relationships. Others come from professional or community-based relationships that introduce you to new colleagues and experiences.

## Changing Priorities

Men's priorities change with age. And, as a man's priorities are the main drivers of motivation for healthy behavior, it's appropriate that the conversation about lifestyle redefinition include an examination of the priorities and changes you can expect. Among men in their 50s, 60s, and those 70+, my survey finds that some priorities rank consistently stronger in importance, while others get understandably weaker, and still a few fluctuate up and down. No matter the direction, when it comes to managing your behavior, it all starts with awareness of change. Of the top eight life priorities men identified, three consistently increase in importance, two consistently decline, and three fluctuate.

## Priorities that Grow in Importance

The three priorities that consistently increase in importance include time spent with wife or significant other, time with children, and time with grandchildren.

### Time Spent with Wife/Significant Other

The increase is most significant between men in their 60s and 70s. Of the men between 50 and 59 years-old, 69% rate time with their wife/significant other as a top priority. This rating grows to 71% among men 60-69 years old, and then by 7 points to 78% in the 70+ age group.

### Time with Children

A similar progression exists in time with children, with the largest jump occurring between the 60 and 70 age ranges. Of the men age 50-59 years-old, 45% rate time with children as a top priority. This number escalated to 46% in men between 60 and 69 years-old, and then grows to 50% in men 70 and over.

## — David —

David is the 55-year-old divorced shipping manager who has been working out and staying active for 30 years. He runs marathons, but acknowledges they are getting a little harder to do. He's adjusting to change:

> I don't have to run a marathon anymore. If I can do a half marathon, that would be fine. Sometimes you're not going to have the same goals, but as long as you're still getting out there, I think everything will be all right."

David is another man who is leveraging his social-behavioral relationships. He has begun to run some shorter races with one of his daughters, as a way to manage the changes in his life, "My daughter and I, we just did the Army 10-Miler. It was nice to go down there and see her. And we kind of work out."

David's other daughter is a 20-year old who lives with him. While she prefers the gym to the open road, they share dietary habits, with Dad doing the cooking, "She wants me to cook whole wheat pasta—but we try to fill something in between, so we usually have, like, a chicken, a fish during the week, and not too much red meat, but a lot of salads."

David is making the most of his situation and doing a great job of working his healthy behavior into his social framework.

## — Bill —

Bill is a 78-year old who still works as a calendar sales representative and is as active as ever. He leveraged a medical event to embark on the course of healthy behavior:

> When I turned 60, I was diagnosed with prostate cancer. And, I guess maybe that was about the same time, too, that my body said to me, "You know, you got to do something. Not that it's going to solve that problem, but it's like, gee whiz, you know. Get out there and move."

Like other men who leverage their social circumstances to improve their health, one of Bill's tactics was to participate in a 5K run with his son and grandson. Bill walked, "It was nice to be able to walk with them. My son and my grandson were running and I was walking, because, with my back, I'm not about to start running at my age."

### Time with grandchildren

The most dramatic illustration of the differences in priorities within the age ranges is in time spent with grandchildren. Men 50-59 years-old are less likely to have grandchildren than men 60-69 years-old or 70+. This certainly accounts in some measure for the low 14% priority rating from men in their 50s. The 34-point rating surge between men in their 50s and the rating from the 70+ group, the largest of all rating swings, has obvious attributions.

Anyone who has grandchildren knows that they are a game changer. Grandchildren serve as a classic model of the dramatic social changes that can occur as you age. The ranking increments for top priority are 14% for the 50-59-year-old group, 36% in the 60-69 age bracket, and 48% among those 70+.

## — Bob —

Remember Bob? He's the 65-year-old fundraiser and Army veteran whose grandchildren live with him and his wife. Bob's extremely active, playing golf and hitting the gym regularly, but, in addition, provides a great example of a man who is proactively dealing with his ability to manage change by finding new forms of fitness. Bob's newest pursuit, swimming at the local YMCA, also strengthens his connection to his grandchildren.

Right now, I'm venturing into a new form of fitness. I'm swimming, distance swimming. Having a lot of fun with that, because I'm setting goals for myself. My young one (granddaughter) is on the swim team at the YMCA, and she is terrific. She's a natural. And I just watch her practices. Couple times a week I'll go and sit through, and it just, it motivates me. It just inspires me, wow, how—you known, how great is this, to see this?

### Declining Priorities

Declining priorities include hobbies and job/career.

### Hobbies

Among men 50-59 years-old hobbies rate as a top priority by 50% of the men, but in the 60-69 cohort, hobbies fall to 43%, and then drop further to 38% among 70+ men.

## — Tom —

Tom is the 78-year old tour guide you met earlier. He offers a great comparison between his former approach to yard work, and his current management and redefinition of this task:

> Well, one strategy is you have to realize you can't do what you did before. And I'm talking at my age now is that— you know, I used to be able to go outside at 8:00 in the

morning and work cutting shrubs, putting mulch down, whatever. And, I wouldn't come in until 5:00, you know, quit. Put in eight hours, sometimes nine. Go after supper and do it. I realize now I can't do that because my knees won't support me that way, and so I break big jobs up into smaller chunks. And so, yesterday, after this nice brunch, I came home, changed clothes, went out, and just worked on the bed that was outside of the front of my house, and that took about two hours, two and a half hours, and I called it quits. And I'm not going to work on the yard again for another couple of days.

Tom gives us more regarding his decision to stop cleaning the gutters and climbing the ladder at 75:

I hired help. I used to get up and do the gutters. I would get a 40-foot ladder and go up. But when I got to be about 75, I said—and the wind was blowing that day. I said, "What are you doing up here, Tom? Better think about another way of doing this." So, I got a gutter guy that comes in now twice a year and cleans the gutters out for me. So, I have hired out—I got a guy that mows the lawn and puts the chemicals down. But, you know, I look at the job and say, "Can I do that?" And if I can do it, can I break it up into smaller pieces? That's the way I approach it.

Not everyone has Tom's resources to deal with his yard and house, but Tom is thinking about his health, and, more specifically, his safety. Most importantly, he's proactively managing and redefining his role.

### Job/Career

The consistent decline in job/career as a priority data tracks with what you would typically consider a traditional pattern associated with retirement in the mid-60s. The downward progression of job/career as a top priority from 47% among those 50-59 years-old to 29% from those 60-69 years-old to just 15% in 70+ is not surprising.

## Fluctuating Priorities

Fluctuating priorities included travel, faith/service to my church, and community service/volunteering.

### Travel

Overall, travel is the second highest rated priority, with 52% of the men rating it as top priority. The age breakdown shows that travel rates as a top priority by 48% of men aged 50-59. It then grows to 54% among men between 60 and 69, and then, perhaps understandably, drops to 52% in the 70+ category.

### Faith/Service to Church

Faith/service to church exhibits a decrease as a priority between the 50 and 60-year-old brackets, but then reflects an upturn in 70+. Receiving an overall priority ranking of just 30% among the eight factors, men 50-59 years-old give faith/service to church a top priority rating of 32%, while the 60-69 years-old group rating drops to 27%, followed by an increase up to 33% in the 70+ bracket. The small amount of variability between all three ratings, combined with the overall rating of 30%, places this factor in the lower tier of the priorities. Nevertheless, the value of this citation is the illustration of the age-related fluctuation and its contribution to the argument for continuous attention to redefining goals.

### Community Service/Volunteering

Among the eight priorities, community service/volunteering is the lowest score, with only 23% rating it a top priority. Nevertheless, the factor exhibits fluctuation among the age-group rankings. Men 50-59 years old give it a 22% rating, which then drops a point to 21% among men 60-69 years old. The rating jumps to 26% in the 70+ category, the most significant adjustment among the brackets. As with the other lower- rated factors overall, community service/volunteering's role in this assessment of priorities is to present further evidence of change.

## Awareness of Change

Awareness is a continuous theme throughout this book. It applies to change as well. The findings on priorities offer one glimpse. They reinforce the point that change is present in men's lives in a material way. Of what should you be aware?

The most significant takeaway is clearly the influence of grandchildren. With a 34-point increase in importance between men in their 50s and 70s, the impact screams out. Of that 34-point move, the 12-point uptick between those in their 60s and 70s is equally significant.

As the leading priority, overall time spent with wife/significant other also requires attention. The change over time is compelling. The nine-point rise in rating between men in their 50s and 70s is noteworthy. With seven of the nine-point boost occurring as men move from their 60s into their 70s, the momentum of the change with age is apparent.

Among the declining factors, the 32-point drop in the importance of career/job is the strongest. It is an understandable shift. Over time and with more study of the increasing number of older people in the workforce, it will be interesting to see if this priority shifts, particularly among more focused demographic cohorts. The question is an important consideration.

Hobbies represent another declining factor that poses questions for further study, but is notable for its movement as a priority. The 12-point drop over the three-decade age span is interesting, with seven of the 12 points coming between the 50-60 age groups and a five-point dip between 60 years-olds and 70+. Intuitively, one would think that older men would have more time and interest in hobbies, particularly as their interest in their career wanes and the relatively higher overall rating it receives at 44%. Hobbies need not be physically stressful, but do pose that possibility. The men in my interviews cite examples such as chopping wood and gardening among their hobbies. Again, hobbies are a point for more investigation and certainly something to contemplate in redefining your behaviors.

As the second highest rated priority, overall travel warrants examination and its fluctuation draws further attention. The six-point increase between the 50-59-year-olds and 60-69-year-olds represents a notable shift in importance. However, the drop among the 70+ year-olds draws equal consideration. The movement is consistent with a theory of increased time and opportunity among the 60-69-year-olds versus the 50-59-year-old cohort and perhaps a diminished physical capacity or interest to travel in the 70+ bracket. However, at 52%, travel remains a highly ranked priority in the 70+ category and is consistent with some of the overall observations in this group about their ability to attain and sustain a healthy lifestyle.

If change, albeit slight or significant, is present in such core measure as a man's priorities, consider the ripple effect into social and health behaviors. Stories from the men I interviewed provide more insights into how men redefine motivations and translate them into their approach to healthy lifestyles.

## Redefining Men

Healthy men embrace change. By welcoming change, they seize the power of that change to redefine their motivators, tactics, and behavioral strategies to enhance the quality of their lives. They tap these same approaches to adapt to the challenges of unwelcomed circumstances. Stories from the men I interviewed cover all these dimensions and run the gamut from new motivators to day-to-day habits to rituals that reflect their adaptations.

Many respond to their conditions by coupling social and behavioral experiences when the opportunity presents itself. Common to all is their ability to maintain their passions for health through their willingness to adjust and redefine their behaviors.

## — Rod —

Rod is a 66-year-old self-employed carpenter and Vietnam veteran. His attitude toward adjusting with age offers a great perspective relatable to many men:

> I mean, I was always—I was always active in sports growing up. I stayed active. I ran. I was a member of a gym for a bunch of years. It becomes more apparent that the older you get that the more important it is to try to be healthy, you know. When you're young, you're—you know, you're immortal. At some point in time, you have to come to grips with your own mortality.

He zeros in on managing change with age:

> I think that the older you get, the more you realize that what you've been doing or what you need to do is that much more important. It's just in general. It's like, okay. You know, make sure you do this. Make sure you get checked. Do this. Eat, eat the right things. Don't eat the wrong things, so on and so forth, and stay active. I think that's the whole key: staying active.

## — Carmen —

Carmen is the 65-year-old retired construction worker. At age 59, he received a diagnosis of thyroid disorder. Before the diagnosis, he took no medication. Since diagnosis, the thyroid condition is under control, but now he's on cholesterol and blood pressure medicine. His healthy lifestyle is, in large measure, his response to his medical condition.

Carmen leveraged the power of inflicted change to spur his healthy behavior:

> Well I guess I used to try to eat healthy—but then when I got sick with my thyroid that changed me a whole lot. Then I said, "Well, this is not good. I have to start doing something a little bit more than what I'm doing." And my wife got on board with that, and that's where I got to where I am now.

The interviews certainly demonstrate how men redefine their behaviors, adjusting to changing circumstances. To these I add two final examples from professional sports.

## — Jamie Moyer and George Blanda —

Sports fans over 50 are likely to recognize these names. Jamie Moyer and George Blanda are folk heroes for their longevity in professional sports. Their careers in Major League Baseball and the National Football League, respectively, extended far beyond the norm. As players, and as men, they defied the odds and won the hearts of American men—and probably quite a few women.

Their inclusion here is simple. Their success ties directly to their ability to adjust their game—to redefine themselves with age. As a result, they were able to stay competitive in a highly competitive field and contribute to championship teams well into their 40s.

For every man who needs inspiration to continue the fight for fitness, who doesn't believe that one can extend good health, well-being, and happiness into your later life, just look at the accomplishments of Jamie Moyer and George Blanda, their willingness to embrace change, and the wisdom of their tactics. They personify motivation in men.

## — Jamie Moyer —

One of the most inspirational examples of a man who adjusted with age is Jamie Moyer. Moyer, who is now 52, pitched in Major League Baseball (MLB) for 25 years (1986-2012). He was 49 years old at the time of his final MLB game, the oldest player in the major leagues, with the most wins, losses, and strikeouts of any active MLB pitcher. Moyer had a remarkable career that I personally had the privilege to witness during Moyer's time with the Philadelphia Phillies, my hometown team.

Moyer pitched for eight teams over the course of his career, was named to the All-Star team in 2003 while with the Seattle Mariners, and won a World Series ring with the Philadelphia Phillies in 2008. A testament to his character and the respect he garnered, Moyer has received numerous awards for philanthropy and community service, including the Roberto Clemente Award, the Lou Gehrig Memorial Award, the Hutch Award, and the Branch Rickey Award.

Moyer's pitching approach evolved with age and his pitching style epitomizes the principle of adjusting with age; his longevity as a MLB pitcher relied on his control and mixing his pitches rather than velocity. Like most major league pitchers, Moyer lost his velocity as he aged. His average fastball was about 80 mph in 2012, a very slow speed. To sustain his career, and extend his success, Moyer threw five main pitches: a sinker, a cut fastball, a slider, a changeup, and a curveball. This combination of control and mixing pitches served him well, as did his determination. Moyer is an example of a man who knew what he wanted, believed in himself, and found a way to do what he loved, by changing his approach and adjusting with age. (https://en.wikipedia.org/wiki/Jamie_Moyer).

## — George Blanda —

George Blanda played quarterback and kicker for the Chicago Bears, Houston Oilers, and the Oakland Raider for 26 seasons, the most in the history of professional football. At the time of his retirement in 1976, at the age of 48, he had scored more points than any other player in history had. Blanda was one of only two players to play in four different decades, and he holds the record for most extra points kicked. He died in 2010.

Blanda signed with the Chicago Bears in 1949, but his time in the new American Football League really propelled his career. In 1960, he signed with the Houston Oilers, as both a quarterback and kicker, and went on to lead the Oilers to the first two league titles in AFL history. He was the All-AFL quarterback, won AFL Player of the Year honors in 1961, and was a four-time member of the American Football League All-Star team. Blanda's already-long career seemed over when the Oilers released him on March 18, 1967. However, the Oakland Raiders signed him that July, seeing his potential as a contributing backup passer and a dependable kicker.

In 1967, during Blanda's first season with the Raiders, his kicking skills helped him lead the AFL in scoring, with 116 points. The Raiders went on to compete in Super Bowl II, but lost the final two AFL Championship games in the 10-year history of the league. In 1970, Blanda was released during the exhibition season, but bounced back to establish his 21st professional season. That season (1970) Blanda, at age 43, had a remarkable five-game run. In the AFC title game against the Baltimore Colts, he became the oldest quarterback ever to play in a championship game and was one of the few remaining straight-ahead kickers in the NFL.

Blanda's achievements resulted in his winning the Bert Bell Award. Although he never again played a major role as quarterback, Blanda would serve as the Raiders' kicker for five more seasons, further testimony of his ability to secure his longevity through adaptation.

(https://en.wikipedia.org/wiki/George Blanda).

## Redefining as You Age

Finding inspiration and staying motivated to live healthily isn't easy under the best of circumstances. Welcomed or intrusive, age-associated change can complicate your life and challenge your healthy behavior. The good news is that there are strategies to help you cope with change and a wealth of information readily available with just a few keystrokes on your computer.

However, I don't just want you just to cope with change. As much as possible, I want you to embrace change and thrive, making the most of what can be a wonderful time of your life. Yes, one can make a strong case that you can thrive as you age if you're open to redefining your priorities, setting new goals, trying new approaches, and leveraging the positive changes.

To support the case that you can thrive, I've cited three central points: lessons from the field of psychology, data reflecting market-driven opportunity, and the positive side of Mother Nature. To this, I've offered real-life examples from men, just like you, who demonstrate how you can find balance and fulfillment in managing both welcomed and intrusive changes.

Point one: Take heart in the fact that psychologists have long studied the process of aging and developed theories on how to manage the changes that you'll experience. You can address physical or cognitive limitations through adaptive strategies built on goal adjustment, with provisions for maintaining psychological well-being. I consider this the management infrastructure of change.

Point two: The fact of the market becoming more dependent on older workers and producing new options for the older worker just bolsters the argument. More than just an economic proposition, employment has social dimensions and can represent a motivating resource for some men. This is icing on the cake.

Completing the triad is Mother Nature's positive side. While she is responsible for age-related decline, she is also a well-spring of life's most powerful inspirations: grandchildren heading the list, but certainly something for every man, regardless of his circumstances.

## Mother Nature's Helping Hand

I've come to realize that Mother Nature provides 50+ men some key benefits that form a context for behavioral longevity and change management that can stand up to the impediments to healthy living. Consider this: At a time in your life when change and the implications of change (most significantly threats to your health) are peaking, Mother Nature provides us the motivational support that comes with age, (i.e. grandkids, time, and money to travel when you retire), to confront them. If men can leverage these motivational opportunities and sustain a healthy lifestyle, they can create the potential for a fulfilling life.

As for the study men, they are a source of inspiration and illustration. You saw how Bob, when faced with a social circumstance in which his two granddaughters were living with him, leveraged the situation for motivation to expand his exercise regimen and take up swimming. Dave found peace of mind moving from marathons to shorter races, particularly when he was able to run with one of his daughters. And, Bill used his encounter with prostate cancer to embark on a healthy lifestyle that today includes walking with his son and grandson. These serve as just a small sample of what men do across the nation, every day.

## Change Management in Five Steps

So, what should you do to maintain your motivation for healthy behavior when confronted with change? How best can you approach the changes that are upon you or those that may arise in the future? What's the key to successfully managing change? I've boiled it down to five key steps.

## 1. Forecast Your Change

Now that we established that change is inevitable, it's important to have a management plan and to think ahead. Consider planning on two levels.

### Level One: Major Change

Level One is the ultimate big picture thinking. What significant changes do you see coming in your life? How do you see your life unfolding? What is your social or family situation? Are grandchildren in your future? Do you have children nearby? Siblings? What are your career or retirement plans? Do you suffer from any serious or chronic medical conditions? Are there any other relationships or factors in your life that might result in meaningful change? These and other questions represent sources of change both welcomed and imposed. Use them to build your own forecast for life change.

### Level Two: Translation to Priorities

Once you consider the potential changes, you need to translate them into the context of priorities and your lifestyle architecture. What do these changes mean? Will the changes enhance or detract from either your motivation for healthy living or your day-to-day routines, rituals, or habits? No factor is too small. Remember the importance of micromotivators.

## 2. Be on the Lookout for Change

Change is not always obvious. It can sneak up on you. There's no memo that says you'll have to change your exercise regimen next week because of an impending problem with your leg. Be cognizant of the gradual changes in life: physical, social, or behavioral. For men, this needs to include a willingness to see your doctor. Often, this seems to be a big problem for men. Overcome a man's inherent resistance to visiting the doc and get yourself checked out. It's the first step in managing change.

### 3. Embrace Change

Your attitude is everything. It makes a huge difference. Experts suggest being open to trying different things, staying in the moment, counting your blessings, and acknowledging what you can't control. Reflect on the power of optimism and work to build social relationships. Similar to the physician visits, men don't do well with their social networks. Women are much better and therefore have built-in social safety nets when it comes to managing change. Men, you need to do the same.

### 4. Adjust: Goals, Routines, Rituals and Habits

With acceptance and a firm understanding of how your changes reconcile with your priorities, you are in a position to amend your personal goals as well as the routines, rituals, and habits that comprise your lifestyle architecture. Tease out new routines and again consider the value of micromotivators.

### 5. Evaluate and Redefine as Necessary

Goals are a continuous work in progress. Establishing goals or amending goals based on change is a first step. Evaluating the outcomes of your goals and making further adjustment is part of the management process consistent with the discussion of establishing goals in Chapter 5. Continuous improvement, refinement, and redefinition are standard operating procedure.

The National Institute on Aging defines aging not as a single process but rather as an intricate web of interdependent genetic, biochemical, physiological, economic, social, and psychological factors. Given these complexities, planning for and managing the changing circumstances of life is a must-have (National Institute on Aging, 2016). Embrace change and redefine.

# Chapter 12 Exercises

Chapter 12 is about the inevitability of change and the importance of planning for change as we age, whether self-directed or imposed change. Retirement, second careers, volunteering, increased travel, and normal life-cycle events like the marriage of children and the birth of grandchildren all represent welcomed self-directed change. Physical limitations, medical conditions, or other threats on your level of independence can bring on imposed change, which can produce anxiety and threaten the lifestyle to which you've become accustomed.

Whether for welcomed or unwelcomed reasons, thinking ahead, exploring new experiences, and considering the possibilities of new circumstances is a good practice, one that can go a long way to maintaining your quality of life.

Like the previous exercises, the following questions represent simple steps to help you to look ahead and get a jump on your future, socially and physically. You've worked hard to get your lifestyle architecture in a place that maximizes your quality of life. A little or perhaps a lot of redesign is inevitable so embrace the process. You'll be the better for it!

Think about the following questions:

1. What are the top anticipated life changes, welcomed, and unwelcomed, that you expect to happen?

2. What is the general timeframe when you expect these changes to occur?

3. How will they impact your life? Positive impact or challenge?

4. What's your strategy to adjust or redesign your lifestyle? What are your new priorities?

5. What opportunities do these changes present?

Finally, it's important to continually evaluate the performance of your strategies and redesign as necessary. Remember, change is inevitable. Do your best to embrace your circumstances and proactively consider ways to optimize your position.

# 13

# Be A Hero

THERE'S A HERO IN you and a healthy lifestyle can bring him out into the world. If values represent a man's most powerful motivations, then the image that best captures the transmission of values to behavior is the hero. The imagery is relatable to men and reinforces the bridge between value-based motivation and healthy action. Heroism's focus on the well-being of others plays to a man's intrinsic instincts to protect and provide, while encompassing all of the strategies I've offered you so far.

Heroes defend a moral cause and help others without expectation or reward (Cherry, 2016). When you find motivation for healthy behavior in your values, and do so consistently, you are advancing the moral cause of health, becoming a hero of health. Furthermore, your actions have a compounding effect. You become a role model to the people you love and care about, raising your behavior to a higher level and validating the designation of a hero.

Heroes are a part of our culture. Since you were young, you've come to understand the role of heroes. Comic book heroes, war heroes, sports heroes, and even the occasional local hero who performs a random act of heroism all convey the same core values. Heroism is everyday people rising to the occasion when the forces of evil or hardship are threatening (even if the evil is losing the big game). They embody all that is right and principled, as they swoop in to rescue those in distress in whatever form. Heroes teach us, inspire us, and leave us feeling good about the world. They play an important role in whatever context they exist. We need heroes.

Growing up, you may have also encountered another type of heroism, what psychologist Frank Farley calls "Small h" or everyday heroism; everyday acts designed to help another human being in need. Everyday heroes do good deeds and show kindness when serious harm or major consequences are not usually a threat (Wakefield, 1998).

Your father or mother, an uncle, a coach, a teacher, or a coworker may have had a significant influence on you that kept you on the right path, offered guidance, and helped you to make good decisions. Everyday heroes play a critical role in your life. They shape your thinking, offer sage counsel, and inspire you to achieve your goals. Everyday heroes make a difference.

## A Focus on Others

Thus far, our conversation has appropriately focused on you: your goals, your behavior, and the benefits you derive by living healthily. Heroism is about the others in your life and the values you convey. As a motivational model for healthy living, heroism bundles all my preceding strategies into a context with a higher purpose. Viewed through the prism of heroism, healthy behavior produces value-added benefits to the ones you care for and love. It enables you to be a role model, a more engaged family man, husband, or partner, a better friend, and, perhaps most importantly, an individual with the capacity to help others in their time of need.

Heroism, as applied here, is a conceptual framework, recognizing that healthy behavior in 50+ men represents more than the metrics of achieved health measures. Rather, it acknowledges that behind the sustenance of a positive lifestyle are traits such as discipline, dependability, adaptability, and compassion. These are qualities that others will spot instantaneously and seek out in you.

Heroism, well understood and emotionally supercharged, is important in the male psyche, making it particularly fitting as a motivator for 50+ men and a key tool in your motivational toolkit.

It supports the endgame and fits neatly within the intersection of behavioral and social factors that influence overall well-being. This endgame results in stronger and more meaningful relationships, experiences that contribute to family histories, and personal development passed to future generations. This is all very important.

Heroic acts can serve as a vehicle to promote behavioral goals like diet and exercise (i.e., the heroism of regularly competing in 5K races with your child or planting a vegetable garden), but you can just as easily leverage them in the social and emotional arena of your life's priorities (i.e., the heroism of traveling with a spouse). And, of course, consistent with blended motivation, heroism shines through magnificently when you combine physical actions with social engagement (i.e., the heroism of walking with your wife). These examples may seem rather nondescript but, when performed consistently, they are huge. They enrich the lives of others and contribute to your well-being. If the little things are what count, then consider these items as major entries in life's ledger.

Being a positive influence to others looking for help is an awesome power. Given the stakes, you might consider it a superpower. In any event, it's the power of the everyday hero, changing lives day by day, and one person at a time. Didn't think you had this power? Think again: It's right there in front of you.

## Role Model Heroism

Nothing communicates, educates, and motivates better than observed behavior. When you exhibit behavioral longevity, and carry out a program of diet and exercise over an extended period, as the men I surveyed did on average for eleven years, people notice. Spouses, partners, children, grandchildren, co-workers, friends, and others will take note. They'll see the bounce in your step and be curious about your habits, rituals, and routines. Overall, your behavior will inspire them. Co-workers of mine, 20-years my junior, humble me by routinely inquiring about my diet as they struggled to lose weight.

What is your job as a role model? Be modest. Be open and honest about your lifestyle. Be willing to share, mentor, and coach. Consider it an honor that you've earned. Believe me, it will be gratifying and humbling. Most importantly, it will fuel the fires of your own motivation to stick with your regimen.

## Blended Heroism

Linking social and physical behavior fits perfectly within the framework of heroism. The stories from the men make the case that being involved and engaging with your loved ones creates long-lasting impressions that convey important social and behavioral values. You'll recall Bob swimming in the ocean with his granddaughters, David running 5K races with his daughter, Carmen walking regularly with his wife, and Bill walking in races with his grandchildren (as they ran). These examples demonstrate the power and the value of their experiences. When you leverage the combination effectively, you become a hero to the most important people in your life. What do you do with this? As much as you can. The point here is that the integration of social and behavioral actions is a stairway to the next level, the heroic level. Use it.

## Spontaneous Heroism

Many of the men I interviewed loved to "push the envelope." Regardless of age, they expressed a willingness to try new experiences if they thought it would strengthen their social bonds or extend their physical or mental well-being. At 50+, openness to new ideas and the willingness and physical ability to try new experiences is hero-worthy and can leave lasting impressions. The experiences can become permanent anchors that stand the test of time in the hearts and minds of your loved ones.

At 63 years old, there is one childhood story that remains one of my fondest memories of time spent with my dad. The story represents the first distinctive occasion that triggered a heroic impression of my dad. It's social in nature and the math tells me that Dad was probably not yet 50, but nevertheless underscores my point about spontaneous heroism. The story could as easily be one of a grandfather and grandchild, uncle and nephew, or volunteer Big Brothers. It's about being heroic in the minds of your loved ones by seizing special opportunities to be creative and build bonds. Further, it's about a man having the willingness and physical capacity to engage in the activity.

## My Heroic Memory

It was opening day for Major League Baseball. I don't remember the year but Washington still had the Senators and Nixon was president, which means I was probably in high school in the early 1970s. That morning, (I think it was a school day) my dad said to me, "Would you like to go down to Washington to watch the president throw-out the opening day pitch?" A bit taken aback by the question, I asked more about his plan. He then proceeded to explain that we would fly from nearby Philadelphia Airport to Washington, go to the game, and fly back that night. Now, we had no flights booked or tickets purchased for the game, but what the heck. I said, "Sure, let's go!" And, off we went. Just as Dad said, we hopped a plane to Washington, taxied to the stadium, and, from what I could see, apparently Dad bribed a gate attendant to let us in to what was a sold-out stadium. I don't remember who the Senators played or who won. I do remember Dad pointing out where Nixon was sitting. After the game, we flew home, all in the day's experience. For a young teenager in those days, flying—to anywhere—was a big deal. Unlike my kids, who flew coast to coast several times as children and went to Europe as teenagers, this short flight to D.C. and back was one to remember. It was Dad spontaneously pushing the envelope and his impromptu actions that left such an impression. He clearly knew how to impress his son and show me that anything was possible if you put your mind to it. His actions that day solidified his number one position on my list of heroes.

Role-model heroism, blended heroism, and spontaneous heroism are but a few of the many categories one could construct of everyday heroism. I offer them as further illustrations of the residency of heroism at the intersection of behavioral and social action. It's a great place to live.

## America Needs Heroes of Health

If there were ever a time when the country needed Heroes of Health and the influence of health-conscious role models, it's today. According to the CDC, physical activity declines dramatically across age groups between childhood and adolescence and continues to decline with age. Of children ages six-11 years old, only 42% obtain the recommended 60 minutes a day of physical activity; this drops to only 8% of among adolescents! It gets worse. Adults' adherence to the recommendation to obtain 30 minutes a day of physical activity is less than 5% (Troiano, Berrigan, Dodd, Mâsse, Tilert, McDowell, 2008).

Let's consider two aspects of this data.

Earlier in the book, I described the plight of 50+ men and showed that generally they do not measure up when it comes to meeting the CDC guidelines for physical activity. This is clearly a segment of the population in need of peer role models for healthy living. 50+ men who are able to adopt a healthy lifestyle have the advantage when it comes to influencing their peers. You have the credibility of being one of them. Think about how baseball's Jamie Moyer or football's George Blanda evoked a special kind of admiration and support (particularly by older men) by competing for as long as they did. While only a select group can experience such competitive longevity at the professional level, the formula is the same. When you exhibit healthy behavior, other guys will notice. You'll inspire them! With less than 3% of adults meeting the CDC guidelines for daily physical activity, those that are among the 3% are certainly the exception to the rule and distinguish themselves among their peers. This is a prime opportunity.

Adolescents are the second example. The importance men place on their legacy and the high priority men assign to children and grandchildren, it's the state of adolescent and teenage activity that dramatically speaks to the need for 50+ Heroes of Health. The data certainly cries out for immediate intervention among adolescents. Given the atrocious compliance to exercise guidelines among adults, it suggests that any positive influence in this direction during adolescence can help encourage adherence to healthy behavior later in life. Convinced? Here's what the experts say.

Economically disadvantaged children are at a much higher risk for negative outcomes later in life, such as dropping out of school or getting involved with drugs. However, some kids manage to rise above these obstacles and succeed despite the odds stacked against them. Psychologists call this concept resilience, and there has been a lot of research done to try to figure out what separates the resilient children from the ones that fall victim to adversity. Dr. Emmy Werner (1995) found that among resilient children, one of the recurring themes was having a positive adult role model.

Another study found that children exhibited better academic performance and had higher self-esteem when they had an identifiable role model (Yancey, Siegel, & McDaniel, 2002). Still another important finding was that the benefits were generally stronger if the adolescent knew their role model personally. This means that a positive dad, uncle, or coach can potentially do more to positively influence a teenager's behavior than any sports legend.

Hurd, Zimmerman, & Xue (2009) also found that having a positive role model even protects kids from negative outcomes when exposed to negative adult behavior from a non-parent. In other words, a good role model can trump a bad one. This is great news, because we all know there is no shortage of bad role models in the world. So, even if you don't have opportunities to interact with young people within your family, volunteer or find some other means to connect to those in need. It's transformational.

## Heroism: A Psychological Perspective

Being a role model and inspiring others, particularly generations to come, or society as a whole, are concepts that developmental psychologists call generativity: the process of tending to social responsibilities and contributing to society in a meaningful way (Sabir, 2015). Some researchers differentiate between global and personalized generativity, but the general idea is the same: using your time and knowledge to benefit others. Research also suggests that not only does this practice benefit society but those who exhibit more generative behaviors, particularly personalized generativity, tend to be more psychologically healthy in later life (Sabir, 2015). You could call it psychological karma.

The desire to have some sort of impact on society is understandable. Personalized generativity, in particular, involves leaving an impression on society that is unique to you. Wakefield (1998) explained how not only do you want to form your own ideas, skills, and values, but you want to see these attributes affect and expressed in the world around you. Wakefield claimed that forming identities dominates the first half of life and the second half involves externalizing that identity, making your impact on the world. This is very much in line with the conventional wisdom that, as you get older, you become more concerned with your legacy. For many men, this specifically involves raising children and making a meaningful impact on their lives, thus "passing the torch" to future generations. There are many ways to express generativity, and one such way can be exhibiting a healthy lifestyle.

Finally, there are experts who have identified the major characteristics necessary to be a hero over the long-term. Among the traits are concern for the well-being of others, seeing things from the perspective of others, competence and confidence, having a strong moral compass, having the right skills and training, positive thinking, and persistence. It is easy to see why those in need would seek individuals with these qualities and how the desire to be there for others would represent a source of motivation for positive behavior.

## Everyday Heroes: What's So Heroic?

What makes the everyday hero worthy of distinction? Why would I suggest that a healthy lifestyle rises to the level of heroism? What's the big deal? Well, whether it's the sacrifice involved in sustaining a healthy lifestyle or the act of coming to the aid of someone in need, the world of the everyday hero is much different from the traditional hero—real or imaginary. However, our recognition and praise of real-life heroes should not be, in any way, diminished or altered. What the everyday hero represents is a unique category of heroism, one with contrasting characteristics and dimensions that are unlike traditional heroism. Here are four factors that distinguish everyday heroism and provide a context for evaluation. When one fully appreciates this context, I argue that the actions of these men fully justify the label of hero. Consider this.

## There is No Drama in Everyday Heroism—and That's Okay

Heroism, as we traditionally think of it, is an action performed in dramatic fashion. Be it in comic books, on the movie screen, or in real life, heroic feats are commonly associated with drama and widespread recognition. However, other forms of heroism that can be equally impressive, although much less dramatic.

Everyday heroes carry out their missions in another world, one very much opposite from that of traditional heroes. On the behavior side, there is nothing glamorous about getting out of bed every day at 4 a.m. to head to the gym. No one is there to cheer you on when you order the vegetables in the cafeteria at work and ignore the dessert station. The nightly news does not report on the fact that you just dropped five pounds, can now lift an extra ten pounds, or walked the dog an extra half-mile. No, the day-to-day activities that comprise the commitment to healthy living are often very personal and even mundane at times.

It's the same for the social acts of heroism. A deep talk with your grandson about colleges, careers, and adult life is not newsworthy. A memorable vacation may make history within the family, but is certainly not the topic of discussion at the neighborhood pub. And, certainly the intervention and referral of a good friend to a drug or alcohol treatment program is a highly confidential matter, known only to just a necessary few.

Rarely found in the world of the everyday hero is drama in the form of notoriety or fame, and that's just fine. Persistence overtakes drama in the world of the everyday hero. The hero acts on his own volition in an autonomous fashion based on the desire to do good and insure the well-being of others: every day, every week, every month, every year.

## Everyday Villains

If there are everyday heroes, then there must be everyday villains. There are. I use "villains" as a metaphor for the multitude of challenges that you face day in and day out. Villains can disrupt your healthy practices and wreak havoc on the people you love.

When you engage in healthy behaviors, you are fighting against the villains. The world throws a ton of temptations and obstacles at you. Restaurant servers push the desserts, bartenders want to pour you a refill, advertising makes the fast food look incredibly tasty, product labeling makes a lot of fluff that's not so healthy sound like superfoods, or a late-night meeting may have you pulling into the nearest fast food drive-through to fix your colossal hunger.

The villains may also manifest themselves in the form of medical problems, injury, and logistical roadblocks to exercise. Alarms don't go off, gyms get crowded, the weather interferes, or your exercise buddy is out of town. There are time villains, weather villains, and broken alarm clock villains. You know them all well.

Then there are the villains that afflict the ones you love. The range is equally robust. The villains of physical and mental health, unemployment, school, sports, divorce, money, and a host of others make men's hearts ache for what they do to the people we hold in such high regard. When you stop to consider all that life throws at you and how it makes you feel, it's likely to get your heroic juices flowing to enable you to come to their aid in whatever way you can.

Your support can certainly include diet and exercise or the motivational planning and execution, which is the subject of this book. It can also encompass the social empathy and counsel to address a child struggling with his or her homework, the couple looking to keep their marriage afloat, the student athlete looking to improve his or her game, the businessman in search of capital to start a new business, newlyweds looking for a home, or someone in search of a job. Those in distress looking for rescue can range from your spouse or partner to a child, grandchild, cousin, co-worker, or friend. The list is endless and the needs are diverse. The villains prey on everyone; there are no exceptions. Those close to you need heroes. They need you.

Lastly, in the real world, it's common for those who would benefit most from your counsel to ignore or even reject your heroic overtures. Unlike the comic book hero whose help receives accolades, real-life represents a divergent path. Complications abound, conflicts arise, and it may take several attempts to get through to those in need. Even when you've positioned yourself with the energy and strength to carry out your heroic mission, people do not always welcome it. Yes, people need heroes, even when they're a little slow to acknowledge it.

## Health is a Long-Term Proposition

In a comic book, television show, or movie, the hero accomplishes his work in relatively short order. Even in real life, it's common to confine a heroic feat to some limited period, like a ball game or public safety incident. Not so with everyday heroism: lifestyle behaviors are a long-term proposition.

By definition, "lifestyle" invokes a long-term, (hopefully), permanent condition. As such, there is no quick fix or short-term turn around. Results play out over the long haul. Now, this by no means suggests that individuals can't see results from diet and exercise in some appropriately reasonable timeframe, and enjoy the benefits of such in the due course of events, no question. However, the goal is sustainability and behavioral longevity. So, it's not just about getting there, but staying on the peak of the mountain of health.

So, too, is the case with the benefits to others. The expectation with role modeling, mentoring, or counseling is that the benefits spread over a lifetime. The children that observe their father exercising regularly and watching his diet hopefully grow up to exhibit these same behaviors as adults. Grandchildren represent an even longer-term play. Younger workers you mentor and Little Brothers or organizations where you may volunteer, all offer various opportunities to instill values of health and fitness or related wisdom on life with differing time horizons for the outcomes. Nevertheless, the opportunity to make these long-term investments and transfer your values represents priceless occasions to impart positive changes in the lives of others. Knowing that you have this chance can be a powerful force. The immediate satisfaction of the comic book hero's rescue may be entertaining, but if you're looking for long-term impact then everyday heroism is the optimal path.

Together, these three factors: obscurity, villains, and delayed impact represent quite a challenge for those who aspire to live healthily and leverage their abilities to help others. This is no easy task and quite unlike traditional images of heroic behavior with the clean lines of good, evil, and immediate resolution.

The magnitude of this challenge, coupled with the willingness to transfer these values to others, warrants hero status. As society increasingly migrates to recognize that heroism is a big tent under which a number of deserving individuals belong, it is my argument that healthy living 50+ men certainly deserve a spot.

## Superpowers and Super Strategies: Beating the Odds

Throughout this book, I've brought you the stories of ordinary men who have done extraordinary things. Combining these stories with the responses from 1,000 men nationwide, I've developed 10 strategies that support a new, motivationally based approach to men's health. When considering the anemic performance of our society as a whole, or men in particular, what these 50+ men routinely do for themselves and others is truly heroic. They have beaten the odds by sustaining their behaviors in the face of huge obstacles, demonstrating the superpowers of these Heroes of Health.

For you, the good news is that these men are everyday heroes and prove that everyday heroism is within your reach. I've laid out the secret sauce of motivation as gleaned from the insights of the men in my research. They indeed have special powers, powers imbedded in their stories and the blueprint for their lifestyle architecture I've provided for you. To conclude, let's consider the heroic qualities that lie within the strategies I've offered and demonstrate the significance they represent to yourself and others.

## Special Powers of the Heroes of Health

### Courage

Heroes of Health have the courage to honestly assess their health behaviors on the five measures of healthy behavior and commit to closing any gaps. By confronting the question, "Where are you now?" in the state of their behavior they build the foundation for their lifestyle architecture.

### Purpose

Heroes of Health stay grounded in their values and their commitment to their priorities, which is their personal endgame. They create a vision for social engagement that turns their priorities into measurable goals answering the question, "Where do you want to be?" By doing so, they provide the motivation for healthy behavior, as a means to reach their social destination.

### Creativity

Heroes of Health create a customized regimen of strategies and tactics that address the important point, "How are you going to get there?" with regard to their pathway to health.

### Teamwork

Heroes of Health recognize the importance of teamwork and never try to go it alone. They use *partnerships* to support their mission and are prepared to give as much as they get from these relationships.

### Preparedness

Heroes of Health prepare for every contingency or roadblock that may challenge their lifestyle in order to maintain *sustainability*. They plan and adjust, as necessary, to maintain their behaviors during vacations, business trips, or other deviations from the normal routine.

## Balance

Heroes of Health understand that it's the small investments—the micromotivators—that can have some of the biggest returns. At the same time, they are adept at balancing social responsibilities with their behavioral ambitions.

## Determination

Heroes of Health are determined. Their approach to positive behavior is diverse and reflective of an individual who recognizes that when one door closes, another opens. Much like their comic book counterparts, Heroes of Health are determined to work through any challenge to their desired behavior.

## Optimism

Heroes of Health are optimists. They see opportunity where others see barriers. While anchored in reality, possibility drives the Heroes of Health.

## Resilience

Heroes of Health are resilient. Change does not deter them. Instead, they embrace change and the prospects of new experiences continue to inspire them.

## It's Your Call

Now it's your turn. Are you inspired to pursue a healthy lifestyle? Does the thought of advancing your most personal and most valued priorities get your attention? Do you feel the connection? Does the thought of contributing to the well-being of others provide any additional impetus to get going? Is all this enough to get you started down a new path? It's your call. I won't tell you that you should live healthily. Only you can determine the proper course for you. Your decision needs to be autonomous for your actions to be lasting. I can only provide some context, what the experts call autonomy support.

The health issue is acute. American society is fraught with lifestyle challenges and cultural mores that affect our health in a negative way. Chronic disease and lifestyle-induced medical problems are running rampant throughout our country, and 50+ men are at the center of the storm. To confront the magnitude of the problem, I've provided this alternative pathway, which starts much further upstream in search of the most powerful source of motivation, for it is my contention that motivation is absolutely necessary and the best foundation for sustaining healthy behavior, as it is has the most significant influence.

By providing this extra horsepower of awareness, I'm hoping to strike a chord in the male psyche to prompt action and sustained commitment. By designing your lifestyle architecture around a foundation grounded in what's most important to you deep down in your soul, my logic is that you will have dramatically increased your opportunity to be successful.

So, before you start tracking your calories or the number of miles you run each week, give some thought to your personal priorities in life and their connection to your health. Performance measures for these value-laden goals include quality time with spouses/partners, travel, hobbies, grandchildren, and the like. These are the social measures of performance for your endgame.

The men I studied demonstrated that they built their success in living a healthy lifestyle from the alignment of their values, motivations, behaviors, and tactics. They understand that healthy living is a means to an end and it ties in with the achievement of their personal priorities in life.

Go be a hero. I wish you all the best.

# Chapter 13 Exercises

Chapter 13 is about finding motivation in the impact that you can have on others in your life, and ultimately your own life, by being a role model for healthy behavior. Your simple step is to answer the questions below. They'll help you refine the plans you've established in Strategies 1 through 9 and show you that you have what it takes to be a Hero of Health. You just need to find it within yourself.

## Courage

1. Have you demonstrated the courage to confront any gaps in your current lifestyle and honestly assess your level of healthy behaviors against the practices of the healthy men?

2. Have you considered how your health practices positively or negatively affect your priorities in life?

## Purpose

1. Have you committed to personal goals that will advance your social motivators and inspire healthy behavior?

2. Do your goals reflect a balanced between social (i.e., relationships) and behavioral (i.e., diet and exercise) actions?

## Creativity

1. Does your action plan for implementing your goals reflect a diversified and creative approach to behavior change that will keep you motivated and sustain your behavior?

2. Do you continually search for new and inventive ideas to sustain your behavior?

## Teamwork

1. Have you extended your social relationships, personal or otherwise, as a means of supporting your behavior change and leveraging partnerships?

2. Do these relationships cover all the areas where you need support?

## Preparedness

1. Have you looked ahead and considered the Villains of Health that are lurking around the corner, waiting to derail your plan?

2. Do you have contingencies ready to confront these villains?

## Balance

1. Do you balance your social priorities with your behavioral strategies?

2. Do you look for opportunities to integrate your social and behavioral tactics?

## Determination

1. Do you proactively confront the challenges to your lifestyle architecture?

2. Is your determination evident to those closest to you?

## Optimism

1. Do you maintain a sense of optimism no matter how tough the circumstances? Do you share your optimism with others?

## Resilience

1. Do you embrace change?

2. Are you resilient in the face of challenges? Protecting and caring for others is in men's DNA.

When you learn that caring for yourself is the greatest way you can care for others, you will truly become a Hero of Health!

## My Closing Argument

Behavior change is personal. As I contend, as personal as it gets. Therefore, it is appropriate that my new model is grounded by intimate psychosocial and emotionally-charged factors that comprise one's social relationships. As demonstrated in the 10 strategies just offered, when matched with the behavioral guardrails of habits, routines and rituals, and further supported by individual adaptations of proven strategies to navigate the aging process, the combination forms a platform for sustainability and all the fulfillment that flows thereafter.

But there's more.

Reversing the failures of our current approaches and the dismal results they produce requires a complementary and supportive environment, one anchored in a broader level of cultural change. As social beings, our individual behaviors are influenced by contextual factors. In the case of men's health, my conclusion is that such a high-level of alignment is present in our nation. A constellation of social, economic and political conditions offers the means to leverage individual efforts and ultimately insure success in our drive for a new milieu of men's health.

Accordingly, this third and final section reviews these broader factors and their link to the welfare of men over 50 who aspire to live healthily. Chapter 14 describes the vital role of women in men's health, and what I characterize as a man's loving constituency. Chapter 15 defines the incentives in play to shape a healthy future for 50+ men's by physicians, health insurers (i.e., payers) and policymakers. I present my closing argument.

# 14

# The Importance of Women

VIJAY CREDITED HIS WIFE as his health "role model." Rod labeled his spouse as the "driving force" responsible for his healthy diet. Gautam's wife regularly walks with him, they do yoga together, and she cooks healthy food. Carmen says his wife is a "big part" of his healthy lifestyle. "She keeps me going on the right path, and I'm glad she does." The voices of the men say it all. Women and significant others play a pivotal role in men's health. Any examination of the subject would be incomplete without them, particularly the socially oriented, motivation-based approach to health I've advanced in this book. Their roles intertwine with their men: husbands, significant others, fathers, fathers-in-law, sons, and others. Their support is crucial. In Chapter 7, I discussed the central role of partnerships in a healthy lifestyle. Though many of the references involved women, their significance compels deeper exploration.

Between the sexes, women are the undisputed leaders when it comes to health behaviors. They make twice the preventative medical visits of men, are more likely to have health insurance and take medications, and orient to health consciousness at an earlier age (Institute of Medicine, 2001). As a result, they live longer and perform better than men perform across a number of health measures. When comparing men's health to women's, Dr. David Gremillion of the Men's Health Network said, "There is a silent health crisis in America… it's the fact that, on average, American men live "sicker and die younger than American women" (Gremillion, 2001).

Perhaps the most significant measure of a women's impact on a man's health is in the studies on marriage. A significant body of research supports the fact that married men generally live longer, healthier lives than unmarried men (Choi & Marks, 2011). While not to the degree of marriage, Christopher Fagundes, PhD and researcher at The Ohio State University, believes that living with your significant other may also have health benefits (Fagundes, 2012).

Best known for their expertise in rescuing men from one of man's most serious afflictions, the healthcare attention gap, women are the ones who schedule the doctor's appointments, get prescriptions filled, and insure that a man gets his screenings. The field of psychology calls women the "household managers of health." They keep their man conscious of changing body conditions and advocate for the acceptance of medical treatment when questions arise.

By all measures, when it comes to a man's health women are a driving force. They need to be. Sadly, on their own, the statistics show that men drop the ball big time. However, by leveraging socially and emotionally anchored motivation, there is hope for men to improve their prospects for self-regulated positive behavior—with a little help from women.

## Women as Motivators

Women also play predominantly as a man's motivator. You'll recall that my survey measured the significance of numerous relationships in a healthy man's life. Highest-rated are spouses, and significant others. On average, 73% of the men I surveyed rated spending time with their wife/significant other as their number one priority. The number increases to 78% among those 70+. Remember also that 76% of the men I polled indicated that their top priorities motivated them and 74% frequently ponder these priorities. What we saw earlier bears repeating. Spouses, and significant others are a man's highest priority and their most powerful source of motivation.

Beyond serving as the wellspring of behavioral motivation, women represent an essential element in carrying out a man's lifestyle architecture, social and behavioral. They are the goal planners, organizers, and travel companions as well as exercise partners, dietary allies, caregivers, and health care navigators. Their support has multiple dimensions and numerous forms. If men's health is a team sport, then women are the most valuable players.

## To the Men, Women, and Those Without a Significant Other

To the men reading this book, if awareness is at the core of my message, then there is much to gain by extending your awareness to include the perspective of women and their motivation playbook. As with any team, each player needs to know the role and responsibilities of their teammates for peak performance. This extends to men's health and in a big way.

To the women, while I hope my research has already conveyed some supportive insights into the motivations of healthy men, here I'll offer you some further observations and an action agenda, based on what I've learned from the men I've researched and their best practices.

To those without a life partner, those that may have lost their love, or may not have a supportive spouse or significant other, I want to open the conversation to you as well. The strategies apply and the message holds. While you may not be in a romantic relationship or receiving a robust level of support for healthy behavior, you can find inspiration and support elsewhere: children, grandchildren, relatives, volunteerism, professional relationships, and other non-romantic social connections. The stories from our men validate this point.

**Kevin**

In the context of a spouse whose dietary orientation background is strictly meat and potatoes, Kevin grocery shops on his own and maintains a vegetable garden with his children as a means to inspire and sustain his healthy lifestyle.

**Jay**

Jay has a wife who struggles with her dietary choices. Undeterred, he has a long-standing friendship with his doctor, highlighted by their mutually supportive healthy dining habits, and regularly shares meals with his daughter.

**David**

David, a divorcee, runs in 10-mile races with his military-enlisted daughter.

**Robert**

Robert, a widower, finds strength in his faith and support for his fitness by walking his dog twice a day, seven days a week.

While the data puts the spousal relationship at the top of the pyramid, it is by no means exclusive. "Loving constituency" is the term I use to capture all those who have the potential to influence and support a man's health behaviors: the women, children, grandchildren, and others who love a 50+ man.

## My Experience with Women & Health Behaviors

Women have influenced my own health behaviors, during my youth and as an adult. I touched on some these experiences in the early chapters of this book. A closer look provides further demonstrations of the effect a woman can have. My time as a single dad also made a major contribution to my health consciousness. Assuming both parental roles created a completely new level of awareness that remains present with me all these years later. Finally, there's my current exposure to health-related responsibilities with my 87-year old mother, which offers yet another dimension to which I'm sure many 50+ men can relate.

## The Women

While I don't have any scientific data to document a correlation between my mother's ventures into the early-stage fitness craze of the 60s and my health behavior today, the fact that I still remember events that happened probably 50 years ago makes me think they were of some influence. Her stationary bike in the basement, the exercise mat, and her various jobs as an instructor in those women-only exercise clubs gave fitness a presence in my life beyond Little League and the traditional sports in a kid's life. Although seeing mom in those leotards was a little weird, never dismiss what a kid will absorb, and how.

Let's fast forward to my days as a divorcee and the girlfriend who convinced me to get a gym membership. While clearly a move to advance our social life, it got me out of my basement, a hodge-podge weight-lifting routine, and the limitations of running outdoors. The move ultimately took my game to a much higher and serious level, opened my eyes to a new world of fitness, and created an entirely new level of commitment to my personal well-being. The relationship turned out to be short-lived, but I'm still at the gym more than a decade later.

Then there's my life today and my wife, Maria. It's a unique relationship. With my background and personality, you already know that I'm successful at self-regulating my own healthy behaviors. There was no need for a lot of support there. I've already described my workout routine. Got it covered. Couple this with a propensity to stay on top of my medical needs, facilitated by a job as a health care executive with access to medical care, and you might conclude that there's not much for a supportive wife to do. Think again. There's much more, and her ingenuity and love provide further insight into the possibilities. Maria has special qualities. She sees what others don't, and she's intuitive like nobody's business. Here's what I mean.

Maria recognizes the value of positive reinforcement and the intrinsic juice of a simple compliment. Her acknowledgement of the fine points of my physique means the world to me (and I'm no body builder). Buying clothes for me that complement my physique moves her game from words to actions. Then there's the research on diet, nutrition, and healthy living. Through her continuous time on the internet, she's a wellspring of information on healthy foods and creative ways of injecting value into our diet and culinary choices.

Maria's impact extends to the social side, as well providing plenty of activities that serve to motivate my healthy lifestyle. She's got it all going, like the trip she organized to Croatia for my Dad's 87th birthday, my 60th birthday party in Las Vegas with my children and siblings, or even our Friday night chill out at the end of the week dinners. It's a full plate of social enterprise, and it means the world to me.

Yes, medical appointments are critical, no question. Support for healthy living, imperative. But rest assured that the continuum of support for a man is a vast and multi-dimensional proposition with plenty of room for creativity and adaptation to your individual circumstances. So, even when you've got a husband who gets up at ungodly hours to work out and watches his diet, there's plenty of other support that can make a huge difference and propel your man to new heights. I echo the sentiments of my interviewees. My wife is an integral part of my healthy lifestyle.

## Health Consciousness Through Role Reversal

My mom lives alone in a senior apartment building. While she drives and maintains her independence, she's had a few medical issues related to her two artificial hips, which cause me to maintain a high level of consciousness with regard to her health and have a very high appreciation for healthy behavior.

On a couple of occasions over the years, her hip has come out of place. This is a very painful and disabling event. Fortunately, on both occasions, she ultimately got to the hospital, and they were able to put the hip back in place. However, as anyone who has been through any type of hospitalization with a parent, you have this, "I never want this to happen to me" moment. Yes, it is reality and, as adults and good children, we do what we must, but if you're anything like me, the importance of preventative health behaviors smacks you in the face as you hang out in the Emergency Department.

Between mom's hospitalizations and the routine occurrences associated with an aging parent, I've become very cognizant of all the nuances associated with health and daily functioning. It makes me work harder at my own health.

## Single Parenthood

Being a single parent is a revelation when it comes to health: check-ups and shots, sports physicals, bloody noses, and trips to the ER. Then there's the dentist, school lunches, and dinner every night. What's that saying about walking in someone else's shoes? Well, as I've told you, the boys and I did fine, but the experience certainly provides you with an appreciation for the importance of your health and, perhaps more importantly, the need to pass on good habits to your kids. With two grown and married sons who practice a healthy lifestyle, I feel good that the effort seems to have paid off. Now I just need to work on my grandson so that, when he is older, he will follow the example of my dad, my sons, and myself in his health choices.

## The Experts: How Best to Influence a Man's Health

Experts have some definite thoughts when it comes to the best way a woman or the loving constituency can support healthy behaviors in men. The interaction between social relationships and health behaviors often categorizes social influence on behaviors in two ways: social support and social control (Cohen, 2004). Social support is any behavior that a friend or loved one performs that encourages or rewards someone for their behavior. In the context of healthy behaviors, this can take the form of compliments on a person's good health or a "good job" following a run (Cohen, 2004).

The key factor in social support is that it is positive in nature and works to reinforce someone's preexisting behavior (Okun, Huff, August & Rook, 2007). Social control, in contrast, involves trying to influence or change a person's behavior. This can be urging a loved one to put down that extra piece of cake or pleading with them to quit smoking when they don't show a particular desire to that end.

There is a good amount of research on the effectiveness of these two strategies to elicit positive health behaviors in the context of a marriage. Many of these studies focus specifically on relationships involving one spouse with a chronic health condition, but it isn't a stretch to see how these strategies can impact daily healthy behaviors as well (Okun, Huff, August & Rook, 2007). However, it is important to note that in these situations, a spouse or others in the loving constituency may take on more of a "caretaker" role. This can have different implications, but also depends more on the attitudes and beliefs of each person in the relationship. An often-studied condition in this context is diabetes. This is a particularly appropriate condition to examine the impact of spousal support because successful diabetes management requires a significant lifestyle change, particularly with regard to daily diet, medication adherence, and daily physical activity.

In a qualitative study examining spousal involvement in diabetes management, Trief, et al. (2003) conducted interviews with couples in an effort to identify helpful and unhelpful spousal interactions. Some helpful behaviors included buying the right food for their spouse when shopping, general emotional support, and reminders to check blood sugar, pack extra snacks, and the like. Some notable unhelpful behaviors included behaviors that involved a perceived intrusion on their independence and autonomy. This is certainly in line with Self-Determination Theory, that people generally require a certain level of autonomy and any actions that intrude on their perceived autonomy, no matter how well intentioned, can be counterproductive.

Another study involving social support/control with regard to diabetes management found that high social control, along with high social support, individuals felt more motivated to exercise the next day, and followed through with that motivation (Khan, Stephens, Franks, Rook, & Salem, 2013). There is also a certain degree of individual variation between couples. In the Trief, et al. (2003) study, some of the behaviors generally described as helpful by most of the couples, were unhelpful to others. The important takeaway here is that what works for some people may not work for others. Therefore, although you can examine general relationships, it is equally important to think about what works best for you and your partner, specifically.

One study that examined possible explanations for variations in helpfulness of social control found that there was a significant difference in adherence for "positive" social control factors and "negative" social control factors (Tucker & Anders, 2001). This means that positive encouragement to choose a healthy meal or go for a run can go a lot further than a negative comment or remark about your spouse's unhealthy eating habits or lack of exercise.

In other words, calling your companion lazy isn't exactly going to motivate them to exercise more. In fact, the same study examined compliance with regard to affective response to the social control behavior and found that the target of the social control behavior was more likely to comply when they felt positively about the comment. If they felt negatively, they were more likely to ignore, or even do the opposite, because you are threatening their autonomy. So, calling your spouse lazy may even make them want to exercise less!

This finding helps to emphasize the point that it is important to communicate and figure out what motivational behaviors work best for you both. Some people may welcome a certain level of control exerted by their mates. What some people consider "nagging" others may see as "helpful reminders" (August & Sorkin, 2011). Therefore, it is important to talk with your partner about how they perceive your involvement in their health behaviors, and to keep the interactions positive. If you each have different ideas about the nature of your roles in each other's constituencies, this could result in unhelpful and unnecessary conflict. It's all about finding that perfect balance between helpful support and autonomy that works best for each person.

## A Balancing Act

So far, I've largely focused on the psychological dimensions of the influence of a spouse, life partner, or significant other. In this discussion, I've offered the sentiments of behavioral psychologists that suggest a supportive approach to behavior change that facilitates autonomous action by the man, as a means to promote his permanent adoption of the healthy practices is most beneficial. A more controlling approach, as a transactional strategy, has slim chances of permanent adoption of the desired behavior. However, when it comes to medical needs of men, spouses and partners often need to be more forceful and controlling.

This is the balancing act. If controlling actions were the only way to get men to pay attention to their medical needs, then many would likely sacrifice the risk of long-term adoption for short-term medical care that could prevent a catastrophic event. Consider the advice offered by Theresa Morrow from Women Against Prostate Cancer:

> The role of women in keeping the men in their life healthy is invaluable. While it may pain you to nag your husband about one more thing, do it anyway. If you recognize any

unusual symptoms in your loved one do whatever it takes
to get him the help he needs; it may save his life.

Layer on the fact that because women live longer than men do,
they see their fathers, brothers, sons, and husbands suffer or die
prematurely. This is true, even though experts tell us that more than
half of premature deaths among men are preventable. All this considered
you could see the rationale for a more controlling approach on the
part of women.

Fortunately, with the Self-Determination Theory psychologists
offer women a means to balance short-term needs with long-term
hope for permanent change. Called integrated behavior, I introduced
it earlier in the book. Integrated behavior recognizes that controlling-
based behavior can be ultimately internalized and autonomously
accepted by the man, thereby increasing the long-term sustainability
of the sought behavior. It's a process and requires an internal migration
of the behavior into a place of acceptance and willful adoption (Ryan
& Deci, 1985). It can be a nice place and very much worth the effort.

## The Loving Constituency Playbook

So far, I've documented the high regard in which healthy men hold
their spouse/significant other, advocated for socially driven goals as
motivators, and promoted different partnership types as strategies.
While I represent the fingerprints of the Loving Constituency Playbook, we need more. What's required to generate the support men
need and fully leverage the strategies I've offered is a playbook for
women that specifically highlight the applications for them and the
other loving constituencies.

The emotional commitment is great. It's where it all starts. Regardless of your status within a man's loving constituency—spouse, child,
grandchild, friend, or other—your support needs to align with the
man's approach, the planning, strategy, execution, and continuous
reevaluation. This alignment forms the heart of the collaborative

approach and supports the team model for healthy behavior. Hence, I offer the loving constituency playbook and six core pillars of constituency support.

The pillars can all adapt to any role in the constituency. In fact, when you apply the same tactics by differing members of the constituency (i.e., the man hears the same message from several people, all of whom he holds in high regard), it is more likely to enhance his overall level of support and decision-making process. He will feel the level of care embodied by the SDT principal of relatedness.

The responsibility the loving constituency must keep in mind is the message provided by Dr. Edward Deci, the practitioners of Self Determination Theory, and other behavior psychologists. When it comes to the health behaviors themselves, don't tell your man what to do: support him and make him aware of the factors that form the context of your support and concern. Let him accept and own the decision to accept.

Much like how physicians outline the various options and consequences associated with medical care enabling patients to determine for themselves what course of action they want to pursue, such is also the case with support and awareness for healthy behavior. As we learned earlier in the book, men are more likely to adopt and sustain the behavior over the long haul if they exercise autonomy in the decision to adopt the behavior. In my interviews with SDT experts, I've come to learn and appreciate the difference between supportive and controlling behavior. The nuances are significant.

The high regard in which one holds the loving constituency gives its members substantial power and influence over their men. If your man's goal is healthy behavior that lasts, then the best influence is to support your man. Influence that spills into a controlling mindset will cause your man to push back and reject the healthy behavior or, at best, adopt the behavior for only a short-term. The intrinsic life aspirations that form the core of my approach are consistent with, and embody, the SDT model and can go a long way to create an effective autonomy-supportive climate, as suggested by the experts. Leverage your social agenda and your common interests. His love for you will facilitate this process. Here are the six pillars of support that comprise the loving constituency playbook.

## I. Acknowledge

Everyone needs to have their feelings acknowledged. The men I've studied made this clear. It's the foundation to value-based motivation and can strengthen the value-stream of inspiration. Loving constituents can lay the first planks in their support platform by acknowledging how the man feels about them and offering a reciprocating message (i.e., you care about him, too, and what he believes in). The loving constituent is a valued and prized priority. The extent to which the constituent has the ability to expressly acknowledge the man's feelings (i.e., as opposed to say a baby grandchild who relies on innate behavior to express love) the stronger the foundation for the challenges that lie ahead.

## 2. Endorse

A healthy lifestyle and a strong social infrastructure supporting continual motivation for that lifestyle is a great thing. If a man shows an interest, endorse it. A constituent's endorsement is certainly a supportive action. More than just a mutual expression of love, the exchange I'm defining is one anchored in a shared confirmation of values and the associated actions that lie beneath a man's interest in healthy behavior. Whether its travel, the grandchildren, hobbies, or the like (assuming it's the case) as a loving constituent, endorse your man's values, the commonality of your mutual goals in life, and the equally shared acceptance that healthy living is a pathway to achieve those goals.

### 3. Determine Your Role

The continuum of support for a man's healthy behavior is wide, so, before a constituent engages in a conversation with a man about their role in supporting his efforts, the individual needs to pose the question to themselves. Use the guidance in the blueprint I've offered for men. You can gain further insight by considering the social and behavioral aspects of the constituent, along with his or her strengths, interests, and aspirations. Are you better at designing social goals and creating implementation strategies that will continually provide your man with a full social calendar that will inspire him to stay fit? Perhaps you're better on the behavioral side? Do you like to go to the gym? Create a healthy diet? Maybe you're all in for the full monte? You'll plan the social calendar, get healthy, and make sure that the rhythm of your man's life maintains a strong and steady beat.

Whatever the case, it pays to be prepared. These important choices and discussions are even more important. Behavior change beyond 50 for men is a tall mountain to climb. A constituent's support is a game-changer.

### 4. Offer Your Support

The loving constituent needs to make the offer, clear and upfront. You are in. This is the team-based message. Take the "we" approach. Your preparation can maximize the value of the conversation, rather than control it. Share details on your desired role. Be specific, no nuance or position is out-of-bounds. And, remember that your words need to be backed-up with actions in the implementation stage.

### 5. Design the Foundation

In this book, I've offered men a pathway to healthy behavior that starts with three basic questions: 1. Where are you now? 2. Where do you want to be? 3. How will you get there? The answers to these questions are personal and value-driven. Questions two and three represent a man's goals, and how he intends to achieve those goals, According to my research, a man's goals and achieving activities are much more likely when motivated by a loving constituency, most significantly his spouse or significant other. This alignment between the motivation of men and their loving constituency begs for a collaborative approach to creating his lifestyle architecture. It's hard to imagine how one would establish any socially or emotionally based social platform without this engagement.

**Where are you now?**

The question requires an honest assessment of a man's adherence to the five healthy behaviors outlined in Chapter 4 as well as his level of social engagement with the members of his loving constituency and others. This requires an honest and realistic consideration of the man's social and behavioral values. You can enhance all of this by the support and participation of the loving constituency. Does the man have any plans to build on? Is there any semblance of a social agenda? How engaged is the loving constituency? Is there any connection in the man's mind between his social goals and health behaviors?

**Where do you want to be?**

This is the goal-setting and planning process. While driven by social goals that represent a man's priorities, it can certainly include health behavior plans for diet and exercise, as well as medically related actions. It includes a comprehensive inventory of social and personal priorities and those of the loving constituency, since they are the drivers for the man's happiness. This can be a fun and interesting process.

**How are you going to get there?**

This is the execution stage, which builds on the plan. Again, the identification of specific social plans, behavioral tactics, and lifestyle activities can be fun. Be sure that your tactics are quantifiable and measurable, so you can evaluate your actions.

## Quality Control

Creating a plan is one thing. Sticking to the plan is another. A key role for a loving constituent is quality control. Monitoring behavior, assessing practices, and measuring performance becomes critical in sustaining positive behaviors. A spouse or other loving constituents can offer insights that the man may not see. It also requires the ability to deliver a candid message ideally in a supportive, positive framework, dependent on where you are on the continuum of supportive and controlling support.

## It's Your Choice

As a woman or member of a man's loving constituency, he values you and regards you highly: You are a priority. This gives you tremendous influence and places you in a unique position to support his healthy lifestyle and an equal opportunity to join in the fruits of healthy living. In this book, I have presented a socially oriented, motivation-based approach to healthy living. Its premise: A man's social, emotional, and personal factors (intrinsic life aspirations) are the endgame and health is a principle means to that end. The stronger and more connected a man to his endgame, the more robust and defined his endgame, the more connected his endgame with his loved ones, the greater his chances are of adopting a healthy lifestyle. Women and life partners in particular, as well as other members of a man's loving constituency, can play a supporting role if they run in sync with their man, whether it's his social agenda, day-to-day behaviors, diet, or exercise.

While men's health still falls short of the time and attention given to women's, the status of men is progressing, and there are tools to support your efforts. The Men's Health Network, a national organization, carries on the work started by pioneers like Dr. Ken Goldberg and others. They offer concrete tips and resources for women and life partners seeking to help men live healthily. The Centers for Disease Control and other federal agencies provide a wealth of information for 50+ men. The bottom line is that it is up to you. The resources are there. I've provided the playbook. With the support of women and a loving constituency, there's no stopping our men from a life of healthy living, fun, and fulfillment. Women and a man's loving constituency can, and should be, part of the man's journey up the mountain of health. It's a team effort. All share the fruits of victory.

# 15

# A New Culture of Men's Health

CULTURE BEATS STRATEGY EVERY time. It's an oft-used business axiom grounded in social norms like purpose, values, and approach (Merchant, N., 2011). Proponents believe that culture makes a big difference. The context enables strategy to be effective. It breeds success. With almost 40 years in management, I wholeheartedly agree.

The axiom also applies to men's health. There are countless strategies for diet, exercise, and personal medical management. Advice is available from numerous sources, from the federal government to individual physicians. Still, there's no overarching or unifying culture of health that's made its way into the hearts and minds of men, or society as a whole. Instead, what dominates men's health is a culture of neglect, ignorance, and apathy. It's one of strong dependence on others and absolute failure when compared to women. We know the outcomes. While they are alive, men suffer much more than women do from serious chronic disease, affecting their own quality of life and the lives of the ones they love. Men die earlier than women do, leaving widows, children, and grandchildren without their love and financial support. Incredibly, men have historically embraced this culture and, through their behavior, passed it along to future generations. It doesn't have to be this way. What I've learned suggests otherwise.

By comparison, consider the culture of women's health and the model of success it represents. Every October we watch the NFL roll out the pink shoes and caps in support of the fight against breast cancer. I've personally run in a Susan G. Komen 5K race on Mother's Day and purchased an official Komen pink tie at Macy's. Talk about embedding into our culture! For many years, the US Office of Women's Health has spearheaded a national effort to promote healthy behavior in women, while the effort to establish a companion office for men seems to fall short on the policy agenda year after year. In no way do I want to diminish the work of many organizations like the Men's Health Network and other organizations that have worked hard for years to promote awareness for men's health. Their efforts have resulted in some important gains:

- Among the sources of programs and awareness activities for men's health are the federal government's Office of Women's Health and the Office of Minority Health (Men's Health Network, 2016).

- In 1994 the federal government, in collaboration with the Men's Health Network, created National Men's Health Week and used Father's Day as the impetus to promote awareness. This grew to the designation of June as Men's Health Month (Men's Health Network, 2016).

- In 2007, the Congressional Men's Health Caucus first established to promote programs and policies that address the unique and challenging health and wellness needs of men and boys and raise awareness of male health issues (Men's Health Network, 2016).

- The American Public Health Association (APHA) created their own Men's Health Caucus (MHC) in 2010 with a mission to enhance the health of boys and men. An outgrowth of the Men's Health Brain Trust/Dialogue on Men's Health, reports that there have been several programs at the state, county, and municipal levels that address overall men's health issues and fatherhood issues.

- More recently, the White House has sponsored a Dialogue on Men's Health in collaboration with the Men's Health Network. The event serves as a forum for education and advocacy.

Even with these advances in advocacy and behavior change, the individuals at the forefront of men's health would acknowledge that there is much further to go. The state of men's health in the US remains poor. This includes the segment of 50+ men.

## A Cultural Context for Men's Health

Nothing occurs in a vacuum and such is the case with men's health. In this book, I have presented the case for a new model of sustainable health behavior among 50+ men. The model emanates upstream from the typical enterprise of diet fads and gym memberships. As supporting evidence, I have presented the opinions and stories of over 1,000 men nationwide, who are both over 50 and exhibit healthy behaviors. To bolster my case, I offered a number of leading theories from the field of psychology, which aligns with the findings from the men. Tapping healthily living men as a source of advice for the 50+ men struggling with their health leverages the inherent benefits of appealing to what I see as a skeptical and tough audience with a messenger of equal status. Once making the case for a social model, I offered a 10-strategy blueprint with illustrations and exercises, acknowledging a man's comfort with a playbook.

But, since nothing does happen in a vacuum, and my ultimate goal is to create a new norm for men's health, beyond my prescription for the individual 50+ man, it is necessary to conclude my message with a reference to the contextual factors that can play a significant role in changing the culture of men's health. These key influencers include women, partners, and a 50+ man's loving constituency, physicians, health insurers (i.e., payers), and policymakers. Together, I conclude, these parties have the wherewithal to move men's health up on the policy agenda in the US, and otherwise support a cultural revolution akin to what the nation has seen in areas such as smoking cessation and breast cancer awareness. The power of these influencers coupled with demographic, economic, and technological conditions present in our society represent a unique confluence of factors that supports my optimism on the ability to make good on such an extreme goal as a culture of health among 50+ men. The alignment of these contextual conditions coupled with a new model for men creates a tipping point for this extremely important dimension of American life.

## Mobilizing the Counter Culture

Fortunately, there is a counter-culture of health among 50+ men. It needs to grow. The men I've studied substantiated my claim that motivation for healthy living is possible when you make the connection between your most important values in life and your behavior. The healthy men have designed a lifestyle architecture with socially and emotionally based goals, relationships, and daily rituals, which give them purpose and a blueprint to sustain their behavior. Moreover, they have fun and heightened levels of fulfillment.

This fledgling counterculture needs to move into the mainstream. Men of all ages, but particularly 50+ men, need a dominant culture of health. There never will be any significant growth in men's health behaviors without a massive dose of cultural change. Men's health needs to be present, constantly visible, and woven into the fabric of society. We need to turn it on its head to make healthy behavior the rule, not the exception. In sports parlance, we need to go from worst to first!

Think about how we convey our cultural norms and how a new perspective on men's health might find its way into everyday life. Can you envision movie and television scripts that portray older men as fit and dynamic instead of pot-bellied and sedentary? How about advertising that presents intergenerational images of older men and young people participating in healthy activities? Or, even a Broadway play that somehow incorporates the social and emotional benefits of men who are conscientious about their health? Sound farfetched? It shouldn't.

What else does cultural change require? Role models for one: Men need to see other men that they respect and have street cred promoting the message that it's no longer "cool" to ignore your health. The days of the caveman are over. Being the breadwinner, perceived or real, does not alleviate a man's need to take his health seriously. The message need not, and should not, be negative. The new culture must scream out to baby boomers, and the next generation of men approaching 50, that health is good, health can be fun, and health is about love and commitment to what's important in your life. This message must be collective and consistent among all our major institutions—government, business, employers, academia, and faith-based organizations. To move the clinical dial, health needs to be cool and culturally hip in order to embed it into our daily lives.

What will it take to initiate such a transformative change in culture? The model is right in front of us—women's health. What women have done so successfully, and what any movement of transformational significance needs, is the engagement of institutional forces that can articulate a consistent message and collectively carry out a systemic social, economic, and clinical strategy wrapped in a culturally oriented message. I call these institutional forces the extended constituency—sectors that have "skin in the game" of men's health, as well as the power and positioning to affect change.

The good news is that these forces exist, they have an inherent incentive to advance men's health, and they're already trending in the right direction. Coupled with these forces are a number of contextual factors, many attached to these institutions, which can serve to "tee-up" a new culture of men's health. It's this alignment of the contextual environment and motivated institutional forces that makes me optimistic about the opportunity to move men's health, and particularly 50+ men, to a new level, one where culture and strategy come together to create a tipping point where change occurs.

## Alignment for Cultural Change

Let's look further into the contextual environment and motivated institutional forces, and examine the case for cultural change. First, we look at the context.

There is a confluence of medical, social, economic, and technological factors present in today's world, providing a wellspring of motivation for health behaviors and the underpinnings for cultural transformation. Here's what I mean.

- Human life expectancy is higher than ever. Between 1975 and 2015, life expectancy for males increased from 68.8 years in 1975 to 76.3 years (Health, United States, 2016).

- While studies suggest that human life may have reached a peak of 115 years, this potential for longevity is attractive. Adding further incentive is a *New York Times* report stating that among the factors responsible for the extension of life expectancy is improved diets (Advisory Board, 2016).

- People are working longer into their older years. According to the Bureau of Labor Statistics, by 2022, 31.9% of those ages 65 to 74 will still be working. That compares with 20.4% of the same age bracket in the workforce in 2002 and 26.8% who were in the workforce in 2012. Among the reasons is the improving health of older Americans. Jobs provide opportunities for socialization, as well as economic benefits. Again, more purpose (The Pew Research Center, 2014).

- Technology supports social engagement. According to a 2016 report of the President's Council of Advisors on Science and

Technology, three common ways older adults engage with the world include social participation, employment, volunteerism, and accessing information and resources. Interacting with family and community groups and being active in organizations can improve a person's health and reduce the risk of disability or death, and technology can assist with promoting such engagements. Social media can enhance social participation with interactive online games, collaboration tools, or websites that introduce people to others with common interests (Report to the President, 2016).

There is a new focus on wellness and prevention. Economic pressure to deliver optimal care, reduce costs, and improve patient satisfaction is what drives it. In health care today, they refer to this as the value-based care model. This focus puts a premium on behavior.

The marketplace is responding with a flurry of healthy products and services. For example, the Campbell Soup company announced its investing $32 million in a company named Habit, which will deliver fresh personalized meals to customers by creating a personal nutrition blueprint based on a customer's biology, metabolism, and personal goals (Walsh, 2016).

Social determinants of health are key influencers within the value-based care model. Clinicians have a heightened interest in social factors that may affect one's health and motivate behavior. Motivational interviewing is one example of the techniques used to examine the influence of social circumstances in support of one's health.

Consumerism in health care is growing. Because of government-led directives to publish patient satisfaction scores and clinical performance measures, the health care industry is under increasing competitive pressure to be more patient-focused. This, along with the focus on wellness, has increased the number of value-added health-care services and an extended attention on behavioral and lifestyle factors (i.e., diet and nutrition counseling).

Population health is a contemporary health strategy that focuses on the health outcomes of a particular group (i.e., men over 50, a city, high-utilizing patients within a physician's practice). With detailed analysis of the conditions of the population, care management and medicine's traditional one-size fits all approach will improve by better tailoring. This bodes well for defined populations, such as men or men 50+.

While certainly not exclusive, these factors represent unprecedented shifts that all point to an environment of change, which is fundamental to, and supportive of, an increased focus on men's health, the well-being of 50+ men, and the social and emotional factors evident in my research.

The motivations for cultural reform are clear: the potential for longer lives of quality, added opportunities for socialization, economic gain through continued employment, the technology to facilitate family and new social relationships, and a total reconstruction of the health care industry that incentivizes wellness, placing increasing value on behavior and offering a number of new services in response to competition. Like a snowball rolling down the mountain with increasing speed and dimension, these conditions will form the underpinnings of a completely new perspective on health behaviors. A range of resources and shifting market conditions are sure to drive culture. At the center of all this change are three major institutions. Let's look at the major players that are there to support you on your journey to healthy living. Happily, their fortunes tie directly to improved men's health.

## The Three Ps: The Extended Constituency

Beyond these contextual factors is the influence of three key stakeholder groups, the three Ps: policy makers (in which I include elected officials as well as the many non-profit organizations and academic institutions, which interact with government), physicians, and payers (otherwise known as health insurance companies). Collectively, they comprise an extended constituency for the health and well-being of 50+ men. Their support, anchored by the strongest of motivations, is their individual political and economic well-being: a value-proposition totally aligned with men's health. An improvement in the state of men has the potential to advance their political ambitions and economic performance. Shifting priorities spurred by political and market conditions have created a universal effort to achieve The Quadruple Aim (improving the health of the population, reducing per-capita costs, and improving the individual and caregiver experience among all populations, including 50+ men).

The result is a powerful incentive to support the cultural reform I've proposed. Historically, the significance of these groups alone would give them a seat at the table. Today's political and market climate increases this significance 10-fold and warrants their recruitment in our mission. A review of the evidence suggests that their engagement is well underway and that there is an increasing recognition that social and emotional approaches are at the heart of these most recent efforts.

For example, in Europe, government-sponsored programs such as Football Fans in Training (FFIT) and European Fans in Training (EuroFit) are motivating men to lose weight and adopt healthy behaviors by leveraging the men's passion for their local soccer teams. At medical schools throughout the United States, motivational interviewing is becoming more a part of the curriculum, as a means to improve medical students' knowledge and confidence in their ability to counsel patients on behavior change. Meanwhile, in the research departments of America's health insurers, studies continue in the search for the best means to motivate healthy behavior in their members and reduce the cost of care, with some studies suggesting that social-based factors are among the most powerful. The common denominator in these examples is motivation.

**Policymakers**

Those concerned with the health of American men face some troubling facts. Four key findings found in a 2015 report of the Commonwealth Fund tell the story.

1. Spending in the US far exceeds that of other high-income countries.

2. Despite spending more on health care, Americans had poor health outcomes, including shorter life expectancy, and greater prevalence of chronic conditions.

3. The US spending on social services made up only a relatively small share of the economy relative to other countries.

4. Public programs, including Medicare and Medicaid, covered about 34% of Americans, with public spending per capita amounting to $4,197 (Squires, Anderson, 2015).

In sum, relative to our international peers, we're spending more, getting less, spending differently than those with better outcomes, and operating with over a third of the costs paid for by taxpayers.

My purpose in presenting these facts is certainly not to trigger a debate on the US healthcare system. I'll leave that to others. What I do want to convey is what many would characterize as a burning platform for change. Within this platform, in a small, but important, way, is men's health. Simply put, as broad national goals go, it's in the interest of policy makers to find ways to reduce the cost of health care, improve outcomes, and find ways to promote health among Americans. Supporting healthy lifestyles in 50+ men, which in turn can put a dent in the cost of health care and improve outcomes, would be a huge win for politicians, regardless of political persuasion. With per capita public spending on health care at $4,197, the approximately 50 million American men over 50 represent a cost that exceeds $200 billion annually. Even an infinitesimal percentage saved through the adoption of healthy lifestyles would represent an enormous savings for US taxpayers.

Researchers Armin Brott, Scott Williams, and Ana Fadich argue that disparities in men's health (all ages) are costly in terms of lost productivity, lives lost, and financial costs incurred by government and employers. Premature death and morbidity in men costs federal, state, and local governments in excess of $142 billion annually. It also costs US employers and society as a whole in excess of $156 billion annually in direct medical payments and lost productivity, with an additional $181 billion annually in decreased quality of life. Their conclusion: Eliminating male health inequities emerges as an important source of savings (Squires & Anderson, 2015).

Furthermore, while the references to social services are often associated with mitigating health disparities, particularly among underserved or poorer populations, I believe that it opens the door to consideration of other nonclinical interventions built around some of the social and emotional factors my research found and their motivational impact on health behaviors (Brott, Dougherty, Williams, Matope, Fadich & Taddelle, 2011).

My argument is simple. Enacting policies and funding programs that support improved health among men 50+ is good policy, and even better politics. I would also argue that the value proposition for policymakers extends to non-profits and the academic institutions who run the laboratories of social change. With a willingness of policymakers to invest research dollars and provide other forms of support to men's health, advocacy, and academic institutions have an opportunity to guide experimentation and advance innovation. Below are two examples from Europe where governments and academics have collaborated to test an innovative, motivationally based approach to improving men's health. While not limited to 50+ men, these experiments testing motivation for stimulating healthy practices are linked to social factors, which can make a huge contribution to the context of our discussion.

## Innovation for Cultural Change

### Football (Soccer) Fans in Training (FFIT)

The Football Fans in Training project is a Scottish-government and UK Football Pools-funded program designed to spur weight loss, increase activity, and promote a healthier diet among men in Scotland. What makes the program unique is the use of teams in the Scottish Professional Football League Trust to create motivation for participation and sustained engagement. The impetus for the gender-sensitized program was the prevalence of male obesity and lack of men taking part in weight loss programs (FFIT, 2016).

By using professional soccer clubs as a setting for a weight management group, the FFIT developers hoped that men's loyalty to their soccer team would encourage them to sign up. Men taking part in FFIT are trained by club community coaches for 12 weeks at their team's home stadium. They receive a program of advice, grounded in current science, on how to eat more healthily and become more active. Men also receive a pedometer to count the number of steps they walk each day (Hunt, McCann, Gray, Mutrie, & Wyke, 2013).

The pedometer proved successful. A study reported in Health Psychology suggested that men would enthusiastically embrace a graduated walking program when the presentation is gender sensitive in context, content, and delivery. Distributing pedometers as part of FFIT was a valuable, reliable technological aid, which motivated men and empowered them in self-monitoring of progress toward self-defined goals. Many men experienced the walking program as a means of regaining fitness, thereby enabling them to regain valued masculine identities and activities, and take a step toward regaining a more acceptable masculine body (Silva, 2016).

In 2011, a research team from the University of Glasgow conducted a randomized controlled trial of 747 male soccer fans aged 35-65 years with a body-mass index (BMI) of 28 kg/m2 or higher from 13 Scottish professional soccer clubs. Here are some of the principal outcomes to note for American policy makers.

- FFIT Retention was high at about 90% at 12 months.

- More men in the intervention than the comparison group achieved at least a 5% weight loss at 12 months and had a BMI below 30 kg/m2.

- A 12-session, gender-sensitized program for weight management and healthy living and subsequent light-touch weight loss support can help men to achieve significant changes in weight, waist circumference, body fat, BMI, blood pressure, self-reported physical activity, dietary intake, alcohol consumption, and measures of psychological and physical wellbeing 12 months after baseline measurement. Mean weight loss in the intervention group fell 5% and is likely to be of clinical benefit.

- Apparently recruitment activities within the clubs has changed men's views about the acceptability of weight loss in men or among their peers and the participative, peer-supported style of program delivery seems to have also explained why weight loss was greater in the FFIT than in earlier trials.

- FFIT succeeded in attracting men at high-risk of future disease, not normally attracted to other weight management programs. Researchers believe that their results have excellent generalizability to other football (soccer)-based settings and have relevance for lifestyle improvement programs for lifestyle improvement.

- Since 2010, more than 2,000 men have attended a FFIT program (Hunt, McCann, Gray, Mutrie, & Wyke, 2014).

The following exhibit contains excerpts of dialogue among the FFIT participants. It demonstrates the comfort that the soccer club setting provides to them, the importance of a gender sensitized, peer-supported structure, and the relatedness produced by the approach.

---

**FITT Participants Discussing the Program: A Practical Perspective**
(Hunt, McCann, Gray, Mutrie, & Wyke, 2013).

*While conducting interviews with focus groups, researchers found that one of the most appealing factors of the FFIT program to the men involved was being around other men like them in terms of age, weight, and supporters of the club. This feeling is highlighted in this excerpt from an interview.*

Participant 5: You could count five points we all have in common, right? One—age. One—weight, yeah? [Club03] supporters, yeah? I've ran oot [out] of ideas on that.

Participant 6: All want to lose weight; all want to get fit.

Participant 5: Every single one of us (overtalking) has sort of, okay, I'll say three, four, five things in common, and that's the pulling thing for the whole lot.

***

*What seemed just as important was not being around a bunch of "Adonises"\* that you would normally find in a regular gym. (\* Handsome young man.)*

Participant 6: I think it was good because it meant that you were going to come along here, and it wasn't going to be like a gym, where they're all Adonises. It was blokes like yourself who'd let themselves go a bit and wanted to do something to get back a bit. And I think that was the clincher, for me that I wasn't going to feel out of place.

***

*What was also interesting is that the men in the FFIT program sometimes likened the club to the same atmosphere they experienced at the pub, indicating that the program created a familiar, comfortable environment for them.*

Participant 1: But things like that was just, and like, wee bits of banter when we're in the gym [at the club] or playing fitba [football] or that—you'd have a wee craic with somebody. And the laughter, when I played football [in the past]—no' at a great level, like—but I used to prefer the training bit to the actually going oot [out] and somebody trying to kick lumps out of you. And that was the environment we were working in [on the FFIT program]. It was almost, coz we had training every week, you know? [Club02_12wkFGD]

Participant 5: It was [like] going to the pub for the banter without [without] the drink.

Participant 1: Aye. (Laughing.)

\*\*\*

*The men also expressed changes in their lifestyles regarding their diet as well. They also discussed these changes with each other, helping to reinforce their positive habits and feel good about the changes. Some of these changes were small, but the focus of the group was on sustainable changes and a mindset oriented towards healthy behavior.*

Participant 1: It was funny, listening to men—and I don't want to sound sexist—but men going on about weighing themselves in the morning and what diet they were on and what they were eating—and I think, and it was good. And there was a real camaraderie about the course.

Participant 3: I don't drink pints anymore, for a start, and that kind of came out, partly came out when we were talking about calories and making you think aboot it. And I'm no ' daft. I knew there must be mair [more] calories in a pint, but I just couldnae stomach the idea of having a bottle of beer while everybody's getting a pint. And I thought, 'Right, I'll try this with the bottles of beer'. And then, once I seen the weight coming off, and that, [...] So, I went on to the bottles of beer. That changed everything for me, because the pints—you're obviously drinking mair alcohol, for a start, so I'm puggled [tired] come six o'clock when I come hame [home] from the fitba. I only, noo [now], have a few bottles of beer. I've actually started taking the car, coz I've got to the point where I realise I'm no ' even needing a bottle of beer. I'll maybe have one bottle of beer.

*** 

*Ultimately, it was clear that putting men among like-minded peers was a key factor in the success of the group. One man likened it to a sort of positive "peer pressure".*

## EuroFIT

The EuroFIT program is a similar effort that draws on the Football Fans in Training Program. The project has received funding from the European Union's Seventh Framework Program for research, and technological development. Much like the FFIT, the goal of EuroFIT is to harness the "love of the game" to engage soccer fans in health-promoting lifestyle changes through their loyalty and attachment to their clubs. EuroFIT engages men through their connection with their clubs to make sustainable improvements in their diet, activity, and physical fitness. Consistent with the FFIT model, the program takes place on soccer club grounds by club coaches (Silva, 2016).

Researchers characterize their work as extending FFIT through EuroFIT's introduction of a focus on reducing sedentary time, physical activity, sedentary behavior, and healthy eating, rather than simply weight loss. The program also draws more on motivational theories such as Self-Determination Theory and Achievement Goal Theory to encourage men to develop internalized and self-relevant motivation, and long-term change (Silva, 2016).

What also distinguishes EuroFIT is the use of technology to measured sedentary time and physical activity. It also provides a game-based mobile-phone app in which players form "teams" to participate in "alternative leagues," which mirrors fixtures in real soccer leagues.

A controlled trial is underway at 15 of the top-flight football clubs in Portugal, Norway, the Netherlands, and the UK. Targeted measures include achievement of an increase of at least 1,000 steps per day (about 10 minutes on average per day, or 70 minutes per week) of moderate intensity (3 METs) activity and an average decrease of at least 25 minutes per day spent expending less than 1.5 MET at least 12 months after their participation in EuroFIT.

Secondary outcomes will investigate whether involvement with EuroFIT reduces body weight by at least 5% at 12 months, if baseline BMI is ≥25, reduces waist circumference, improves eating habits, reduces blood pressure at 12 weeks, and reduces risk of cardiovascular disease, as measured by blood-based biomarkers in 12 months. Also, if it increases positive affect and self-esteem, and improves quality of life at 12 weeks and 12 months, and it has the potential to provide a cost-effective use of resources.

The design of the project allows for widespread replication in different countries, communities, and settings (Silva, 2016).

### Would Team Loyalty Motivate American Men?

Motivation for participation is at the heart of both FFIT and EuroFIT. In both examples, European governments have seen the value of funding these experiments. Based on the initial results of FFIT, there appears to be promise in such unique, motivationally based approaches.

Would such program work in the U.S.? Could you see the National Football League or Major League Baseball developing programs for American men? Is NFL, MLB, or other sports franchises of such significance in the lives of American men that a US version of FFIT would produce similar rates of participation and improved health? Would our federal government fund a program of this type?

Over the past several years, the Men's Health Network has collaborated with several National Football League clubs to promote awareness of men's health issues. The teams have included the Seattle Seahawks, Cleveland Browns, and Washington Redskins (Men's Health Network, 2016). The Denver Broncos and the University of Colorado Health Center have participated in a program created by the Movember Foundation, a charity that advocates for men's health globally. The organization is known for getting men to grow mustaches (as well as women and children to sport fake mustaches) during the month of November as a means of drawing attention and raising funds to fight diseases that commonly affect men such as prostate cancer, testicular cancer, and heart disease (Movember Foundation, 2016).

The NFL programs appear to orient largely to screening and awareness and do not approach the rigor of either FFIT or EuroFit. Nevertheless, the preliminary results from FFIT provide hope that such motivation-based approaches to men's health within the framework of a public-private partnership deserve some serious consideration from American policymakers. The underlying health conditions of the European men do not appear to be very distant from their American counterparts.

Similarly, the men's strong affiliation for their soccer teams in many ways mirrors American football loyalties and those we see in other major league sports in the US. The increasing engagement of NFL franchises in men's health advocacy and screening offers further evidence of a trend for these clubs to be conscious of their fan base and some real and significant issues confronting that base. The FFIT and EuroFit models are worthy of consideration by American policymakers, as they grapple with some daunting challenges to the health of the people they represent. Innovative approaches like these demonstrate the power of socially anchored motivation.

## Physicians

The second of the three major stakeholders are physicians and the health systems that in many cases employ them (it's important to note that many physicians today work full-time for a health system and not part of an individual practice or practice group). Under health care reform and the previously mentioned value-based model of health care, many physicians now have an economic stake in the treatment and clinical outcomes of their patients. The Medicare Access and CHIP Reauthorization Act of 2015 (MACRA) establishes performance measures that will influence physician payments for Medicare patients.

In the healthcare world, the actions of the federal government and Medicare often mirror the commercial insurers, so major directional changes like MACRA become bellwethers for the industry as a whole. The establishment of payments tied to performance represents a major shift in healthcare's economic model and more directly vests physicians with "skin in the game" of medicine. Their economic well-being now directly ties to the clinical outcomes of their patients. Most experts also agree that politics aside, some form of incentive-based payment models will be a part of medicine's future in one form or another.

This new economic model has, in turn, spurred new clinical approaches. Prevention and wellness have become more significant. Behavior and integrated care (i.e., medicine and behavioral health) take on new importance as a means to treat patients with complex conditions. Patient stratification within a physician's practice or defined population becomes key to medical management (i.e., categorizing patients based on their level of medical complexity and tailoring clinical interventions based on their classification vs. a one-size-fits-all model). Electronic medical records become essential to these new clinical dynamics, as does team-based care where nurses, medical assistants, and technical support staff take on new roles in patient management that doesn't require the physician's direct involvement with the patient. What does all this mean to a 50+ guy? A lot.

Economically, the better you do as a patient, the better the doc or his/her health system will do as a provider. Therefore, over time, they will likely be more concerned with what's going on in your life and how it might impact your health, and maybe even ask you! Your primary care doctor can gain knowledge regarding community resources for health, fitness, and social services, as s/he promotes preventative diet, exercise, and your general well-being. They call this the "Medical Neighborhood. For patients in general, and 50+ men in particular, the health care system in America is migrating to a more patient-centered model. With this will come new opportunities for 50+ men to be more engaged in their health, share the values that drive your behavior, and help the clinicians who treat you understand what makes you tick.

One way to implement the value-based model is though something I've referenced several times in this book, and that's motivational interviewing, a method designed to understand and engage a patient's intrinsic motivations in an effort to change their behavior and improve their health outcomes. As I cited early in the book, in my reference to my late father-in-law Dr. Iula, motivational interviewing is getting to know the patient on a more personal basis, using that knowledge to facilitate their treatment, and positively influence their behavior. This approach ties directly to the socially driven approach that are the subject of both this book and the findings of the healthily living men I studied. What's significant now are the financial incentives for physicians and health systems to engage in this activity. Now, a good doctor cares because of his/her intrinsic motivation to care for your well-being, your life, and how your lifestyle affects your health. It's nice to know that Uncle Sam has created a financial model to further encourage further physicians to take interest in such topics.

Another big change in health care is consumerism and new tools that support patient education and choice. Health systems today must measure patient satisfaction through the administration of surveys. You may have received one after your last visit to the doctor. The results of these surveys show how patients scored their doctors and health care providers. They publish the information in your local newspaper and they're available on-line. What is the point? They rate the health systems and doctors on a number of factors. Among them is how you feel about your treatment. Because of these new practices, things like courtesy and respect become increasingly important and support a much more patient-centered approach to care delivery. This means more incentives to offer you a good experience, one that has the power to reduce hesitation on the part of the men seeking care.

## Views from the Front Lines

To explore further the constituency of physicians, I spoke to two doctors with unique insights into the treatment of 50+ men. Their reflections speak volumes about the culture of men's health, but their insight also provides the kind of hope that flows from understanding. Their wisdom offers 50+ men and all patients the promise that physicians are beginning to see them for the whole person that they are, recognizing that social and psychological factors that are critical to treatment, and that motivation for healthy behavior exists outside the exam room.

## — A Genius in Camden, NJ —

Dr. Jeffrey Brenner is a 47-year old family medicine physician who practiced medicine in Camden, New Jersey for 11 years before he embarked on the creation of the Camden Coalition of Healthcare Providers over 10 years ago. His personal mission of innovation and passion to bring healthcare to underserved residents of Camden earned him the prestigious Mac Arthur Genius Award in 2013. I have had the privilege of serving on the Board of Directors of the Coalition and working with him through our mutual employer.

Jeff's work epitomizes what I have referenced previously as population health. In his case, the targeted population is the city of Camden, New Jersey, a city most recently on the rise after decades of poverty and decline. Jeff has organized all the healthcare providers in the city into a well-coordinated effort to challenge the one-size-fits-all approach to health care. By identifying the "frequent flyers" (those with extraordinary large number of emergency room visits) and supplementing traditional medical care with a range of wrap-around social and clinical support services, Jeff and the coalition have created a model that has received national recognition. What does Jeff think about 50+ men and their health?

For starters, he treated many of them and, as he put it, "I saw them committing suicide slowly." He explained how he saw men have stroke after stroke because of factors that were entirely preventable. He also witnessed their wives becoming caretakers and confirmed the fact that "guys don't talk," referring to their unwillingness to share what's on their minds.

Jeff's advice for 50+ men is just what you might think. Relationships and social networks are key. The more isolated you are, the worse your health. He places a good number of men he treated in the dismissive or avoidant category of attachment style. They sought a high level of independence, sometimes avoided attachment altogether, and denied needing close relationships. This included their physician. It is this avoidance of health care and dismissiveness of its importance that has plagued men for years (Bartholomew & Horowitz, 1991).

Where's the hope? It's in Jeff's willingness to confront his own profession and suggest to me that 80% of health is attributable to psychology and social factors. He goes on to question why we expect doctors to be behavioral psychologists and that a culture of health will not be the result of hiring more physicians, but by a greater focus on those psychological and social determinants. Jeff's comments caused me to reflect on the men I interviewed, not necessarily their physical health, which qualified them for the interview, but their psychological well-being that came across to this non-clinician. It was clear in almost all the interviews that these healthy men were, at least in part, healthy because of their social influences and the resulting psychological well-being.

## — A Physician-Psychologist —

Dr. Geoffrey Williams is both a medical doctor and a psychologist at the University of Rochester Medical Center. Geoff, who is 59 years old, earned his PhD in psychology at the University of Rochester where he became associated with Dr. Ed Deci and Dr. Richard Ryan, the founders of Self-Determination Theory (SDT). Geoff is the health care specialist among the SDT crew in Rochester.

His medical practice centers on lifestyle management, including tobacco dependence, cardiovascular risk reduction, hypertension, cholesterol, diabetes risk reduction, weight loss, and nutrition. He incorporates his training in psychology into his practice and is a big proponent of intrinsic motivation and the tenants of SDT, most notably autonomy.

I first introduced myself to Geoff at the 2016 Self-Determination Theory conference in June of that year and was fortunate enough to interview him in August back in Rochester, and then by phone again in September. To get the full-experience of what Geoff does, when I went to Rochester to interview him, I also saw him as a patient. Many of Geoff's patients are 50+ men and his extensive personal interview is quite interesting. As a physician also trained in psychology, he is the exception. He is a physician who willingly incorporates social, emotional, and psychological elements into his medical care.

During the interviews, Geoff explains that he puts a premium on intrinsic motivations and autonomous decision-making. He makes it clear to me that he wants his patients to independently decide to change their behavior. He gears his counsel, accordingly, with an explanation of a patient's condition, the likely causes of the condition, the risks, and the behavior changes he recommends to address the patient's problems. He consciously stops short of a controlling conversation, dictating a course of action or leveraging the inherent authority of his status as a physician. He wants the patient to reflect on his counsel, consider the consequences offered by him, and decide what to do on their own.

When necessary and appropriate, Geoff delves into social and emotional topics and integrates values into the discussion. Goals are a big part of his approach, but he concedes that getting his patients, including the 50+ man, to buy into behavior change is a challenge.

When I ask about other physicians and their level of interest in intrinsic motivation or the psycho-social-emotional aspects of medical care, he indicated that they are "not real interested," but they do appreciate the results he achieves, citing surgeons and oncology physicians whose patients he helps to stop smoking.

Finally, Geoff points out that there is an important message for public health officials in his approach to medicine, a message grounded in his psychological training. "Policymakers should put out a message that is supportive versus controlling; stay away from a controlling message." He cites many of the pronouncements of the Centers for Disease Control (CDC) as too controlling. A more realistic message, he suggests, focused on how alcohol affects your life would be more effective than simply telling people to quit drinking.

During my exam, I got a firsthand look at the process in action. He spent quite a bit of time asking me about my life, family, siblings, and goals. He was careful to let me talk while he took notes. In advance, he'd reviewed my blood-test results, which I had forwarded. He also asked me about my diet, exercise, and personal habits. While happy with my weight, diet, and exercise routine, he pointed out some dietary no-no's and clarified some misnomers for me on nutritional labeling. He explained to me that the coconut milk I'd been putting in my coffee and my oatmeal has too much saturated fat, and that the associated calories from the fat are a problem over the long-term.

Then we get to a more serious topic. While my lab work is good, he says I have prehypertension or hypercholesterolemia and that my ten-year risk for CAD (coronary artery disease) is greater than 5 (the new CDC standard since 2013). Long story short, he recommends a light statin. He plays on my perfectionist tendencies, so I say I'll discuss his findings with my regular primary care physician and then decide. Fast forward, I'm back home with my doc, who has read Williams' report. I've gotten a new set of blood tests to confirm my numbers. We discuss the pros and cons. I now take a light statin, so my heart should be good for when I'm 80. Nothing else has changed in my diet or exercise routine.

The take-away is that Geoff's approach to medicine is the exception. He blends medicine with behavior in search of better health outcomes. His strong reliance on autonomous adoption of healthy behavior may cause some to scratch their heads, and perhaps some wives to reject this theory, but it's certainly based on what he truly believes is the best approach for long-term, sustained healthy behavior. The SDT proponents could point to numerous studies that bear this out.

To me, the interesting message found in the stories of both Jeff Brenner and Geoff Williams is that their motivation for serving their individual populations (Camden City for Brenner and those in serious need of behavior change for Williams) is not monetary compensation but rather a more intrinsic motivation. They both have a profound focus on behavior and the social and psychological aspects of health driven by a desire to affect positive change. Both embarked on their paths well in advance of health care reform and the monetary incentives associated with it. Time will determine which approach proves to be more effective or whether both can co-exist in a complementary fashion. Regardless, both the macrochanges effectuated by health care reform to incentivize a concern for the social-emotional elements of health, and the efforts of physicians like Drs. Brenner and Williams, bode well for 50+ men and their ability to design a lifestyle architecture that gets them on a path to sustained health.

## The Insurance Companies (Payers)

Commercial health insurers work hard to influence positive health behaviors. They should; it is in their best interest. The equation is simple: improve health, reduce medical claims, and make more money. This value-proposition preceded health care reform. With health care costs approaching 17.8% of GDP (gross domestic product), the economic pressure is greater for insurers to hold down premiums and find ways to reduce underlying medical costs (Centers for Medicare & Medicaid Services, CMS.Gov 2016).

As part of their business operations, insurers know what segments of the population require the greatest amounts of medical care and generate the most costs. They know that older men with a preponderance of chronic conditions are likely to consume a disproportionately higher amount of care, despite their reluctance to seek out care. In fact, the deferral of lower-costing primary care can often lead to more costly specialty care when conditions go untreated.

Furthermore, the insurers know that individual behavior has the greatest influence on health, so they're constantly researching the most effective ways to stimulate healthy behavior among their members, and 50+ men are no exception. With strong economic motivations and an eye on behavior, insurers are an important player and a formidable institution in the extended constituency of 50+ men. They have a platform to advocate change and are in a position to examine, test, and extend the research on the socially oriented and motivationally based approaches that form the basis of this book.

The nation's largest insurers, such as United, Kaiser Permanente, and Anthem, have advanced research capabilities and relationships with academic institutions, which give them the wherewithal to focus on men's health. Other insurers have similar resources, as well as advertising and marketing budgets enabling them to fund campaigns designed to inform and motivate healthy behaviors. Historically, payers have focused on more narrow issues of utilization and wellness: requiring pre-authorization for certain procedures, waiving co-pays for an annual visit to a primary care physician, offering reimbursements for health club memberships, providing calls from wellness coaches, and a sending a plethora of literature in the mail. Robust websites, retail sites, and online member services have added to these more traditional responses to cost control and promote member health. However, there are signs that insurers are beginning to recognize the potential beneftis of the socially based approaches to health, setting the table for deeper examinations of the psychology behind the motivation for health behavior.

### Searching for Motivation for Healthy Behavior

Aaron Smith-McLallen is a research scientist at Independence Blue Cross (IBX) in Philadelphia, a major health insurer in Southeastern Pennsylvania. He was previously at the University of Pennsylvania, where he was a post-doctoral research fellow after earning his PhD in philosophy and social psychology from the University of Connecticut (Smith-McLallen, 2013). I sought out his reaction to my research. Turns out, he's very much interested in social motivators as drivers of behavior.

Smith-McLallen shared a meta-analysis of health behavior he had conducted and his insights into improving health outcomes (Smith-McLallen, 2015). Two points jump out from his report as relevant to my research. First, he cites a 2006 study (Webb & Sheeran, 2006) pointing out that social encouragement, social pressure, and social support are among the top-rated behavior change methods. Social factors receive the second highest rating among 17 intervention characteristics. Second, Smith-McLallen focuses on an Integrated Model of Behavior Prediction (IM), which includes a number of points that build on social relationships and reinforce my survey findings from the healthy men. These include:

- Leveraging social norms, social relationships, and subjective norms.

- What others who are important to you want you to do.

- What are others doing?

- Who are the people who would be supportive of or approve of you walking 30 minutes a day, at least five days a week for the next eight weeks?

- Social relationships have positive impacts on health.

- Provide emotional and instrumental support: caring, acceptance, encouragement, and practical assistance.

- Understand that a lack of social relationships and social support is detrimental to health.

He also cites the importance of familiar factors that can help his members overcome interruptions in the intention-behavior relationship. Among them are humor, commonality, and social consensus; interestingly, factors just seen in the men who participate in the FFIT program.

Smith-McLallen's research provides direct evidence of an insurer's interest in finding motivation for healthy behavior. While not exclusively geared to 50+ men, the work is nevertheless indicative of investments taking place in such pursuits and increasing the place of social, emotional, and psychological factors in the sphere of motivation research. Smith-McLallen's analysis suggests that more narrowly directed efforts for 50+ men are not outside the realm of possibility, when considered in the context of its economic value proposition.

## Leveraging the Confluence for Cultural Transformation

Yes, timing is everything, and there is a combination of factors creating a tipping point for a new culture of men's health, and, within this transformation, the prospect for improved health of 50+ men. The burning platform is set. It includes essential pillars, such as economic, political, social, and clinical motivation and the adjoining alignment of the institutions of implementation: policymakers, physicians (health care providers), and payers (the insurance industry). Moreover, the model is there in women's health. What remains is the lift to a more prominent place on the nation's policy agenda for men's health. What will this lift take? Both culture and strategy.

Culture takes shape by messaging, which permeates all facets of society but requires backing by strategy. As a society, we need to understand fully the horrid state of men's health, our ability to make dramatic change, and the consequences of failure. Men's health needs to come off the back burner and turn from an afterthought to something that's continually present in the eyes of society. Smoking offers a case study that demonstrates how combining culture and strategy transforms behavior.

The prevalence of smoking in the United States declined among men from 57% in 1955 to 23% in 2005 and among women from 34% in 1965 to 18% in 2005. A multi-pronged public-private sector effort started in 1964 with a report from the US surgeon general, followed by other reports documenting tobacco's health effects, including the effects of secondhand smoke (Schroder, 2007). Over time, this led to a number of actions to limit smoking in various venues—first on airplanes and through the actions of state and local governments in a wide range of public buildings, campuses, stadiums, and other public, and ultimately privately-operated spaces such as restaurants. Fueling these movements were limitations on advertising (i.e., television, billboards), tobacco education in schools, and smoking cessation programs administered by public health agencies. Proactive messaging, both government-sponsored and privately sponsored, reinforced the negative images of smoking and accentuated the positive benefits of quitting.

Private employers followed suit by establishing smoke-free workplaces and designated smoking areas. The overarching effort that transformed smoking was a cultural phenomenon. It changed how society viewed smoking from something perceived as "cool" and socially appropriate to something perceived by many as unhealthy and disgusting. Statistics show that even today many smokers wish they could quit.

Tobacco is an example of cultural and strategy working hand in hand. The genesis was governmental but, true to form of most transformations, the culture as a whole ultimately absorbed it into all facets of life.

Policymakers could do the same for men's health. Whether supporting the Americanization of programs like FFIT, creating a federal Office of Men's Health, or promoting men's health through public service messaging, there is a wide range of policies that could initiate cultural reform and begin to heighten the public's awareness of the tremendous shortfalls and consequences suffered due to a lack of attention. The same holds true for state and local governments.

Local partnerships between health care providers and municipal and county officials can build cultural reform at a grassroots level. Wouldn't it be great if every primary care physician, as well as specialists, were fully aware of all the parks, running tracks, and public fitness programs in their town or county (one of my own pet peeves)?

Most important is messaging these strategies in a way that's not only data driven but socially linked. As the healthy men exhibited, a strong link between behavior (the means) and the social and emotional outcomes of healthy behavior (the ends) represent some of the strongest motivators for men. Images portraying the benefits of a man's behavior, whether representing longevity or the ability to engage socially, can be part of public service campaigns headed by spokespersons who further drive home the message. Moreover, public health initiatives, at all levels of government, need to incorporate their own version of the socialization of men seen in the FFIT program, finding common bonds that build enthusiasm for healthy behavior.

Physicians and health systems can enhance their use of motivational interviewing and acknowledge the value of social determinates for what they would characterize as patient compliance or adherence. Focusing on intrinsic motivators and establishing patient protocols that capture these factors in the first place would be a big step further. The approaches of physicians like Dr. Brenner and Dr. Williams need to become more commonplace and less the exception. Integrated medical-behavioral models that build on social-emotional factors can go a long way in this effort.

Finally, insurers have an opportunity to join with their institutional cohorts and mirror the social-psychological approach by advancing behavioral and motivational research on men, and 50+ men in particular. Building on and incentivizing the socialization so important to men, and exhibited in the work of Dr. Smith-McLallen, would represent an entirely new approach for them. Public-private partnerships created around these social models could represent the breakthrough programming for which they have been searching.

These and many other actions on the part of policymakers, physicians, and payers are at the heart of cultural reform, because, at its core, transformation needs drivers: institutions with common motivations, talent, and resources. For too long men have fallen short when it comes to their health. The wait must end. It's time.

# Epilogue

IT'S SATURDAY DECEMBER 17, 2016, and I have just returned from the gym. I'm at the kitchen table reading the papers over breakfast, and my eyes land on a promo on the header of the *New York Times* Arts & Leisure Section of Sunday's paper (which I receive on Saturday) highlighting a story on Tony Bennett. The prior Saturday night we'd taken my 90-year-old dad to see 90-year-old Bennett in concert at nearby Rowan University as a pre-holiday treat and fun night out, so I was curious as to what the article said. I wanted to see if it matched our recent experience with the entertainer.

For us, Bennett was amazing. The concert was 90 minutes of non-stop vocals with a voice that sent chills up our spines and had our feet tapping in rhythm. Interspersed throughout the performance were probably three or four standing ovations, which appeared to inject more and more energy into Bennett as the night went on. His repertoire of hits and American standards clearly struck a chord with my dad and the entire audience. He was engaging, sharp, and had a presence that we felt throughout the theater. What a show.

The *Times* article not only confirmed that Bennett is a very special person but provided a great illustration of a man who manages the marathon of life with art and skill and is energized by the fulfillment that he derives. The context of the piece by John Marchese was an upcoming television special "Tony Bennett Celebrates 90: The Best Is Yet to Come" pointing out that his status as an American legend prompted network executives to give the 90-year-old's special a two-hour time block, a rare occurrence last extended to Bob Hope at 93 (Marchese, 2016). The article chronicles Bennett's life, including his struggle with drugs and alcohol, as well as his climb back into pop culture, through appearances on MTV and later in recording with contemporary singers, most notably Lady Gaga, with whom he became the oldest living performer to have a number one album.

Finally, Marchese describes what he characterizes as Bennett's "voracious curiosity," which included starting piano lessons and a penchant to improve on his longstanding passion for painting, by devoting time daily. These personal ambitions are in addition to a career that remains in full-gear: a new book just published entitled appropriately "Just Getting Started," more albums, and 30 concert dates on his schedule for the first half of 2017.

Bennett's opening act that night was his daughter, Antonia, and since 1979, his son, Danny, has managed his career. In separate interviews, Bennett has attributed his health and ability to continue performing to his wife. "I also have a wonderful wife, Susan, who makes sure I eat healthy every day, and I work out at least three times a week," he said (Pensiero, 2016).

Without question, Bennett is an inspiration for us all. He touched my dad that night and, in the process, sent me a message. For as much as Bennett inspires, he also illustrates a man employing the strategies I've offered, blending them artfully into a melody of behaviors that form the cornerstones of lifestyle architecture. Here's what I mean.

First, let's look at the close relationship he maintains with his family. His daughter is singing with him, his son manages his career, and his wife is at his side, tending to his diet and exercise regimen. He epitomizes the blending of social-behavioral action, drawing both motivation and support from a well-defined loving constituency with a woman at the center. The illustration continues with a strong argument that his fans are part of his loving constituency and a unique form of inspiration, as I witnessed on that December evening.

Next, think about Bennett's ability to reclaim his life from adversity, in his case, addiction. His evolution reflects a personal dexterity to adjust and evolve that has fueled a professional comeback of enormous proportion. He is the master of change and diversification, teaming up with contemporary artists such as Lady Gaga, resulting in huge success. This capacity extends into his personal life, where he's starting piano lessons and is relentless about his passion for painting. As if that wasn't enough, the man still maintains a very respectable work schedule.

So yes, at 90, Tony Bennett remains an extraordinary entertainer, but there's so much more men can learn from his story. Bennett is a man who has found motivation in his life's priorities. Coupled with an approach to life that embraces change and new experiences, Bennett's motivation has enabled him to maintain an active life and a level of well-being that was evident in his performance. He personifies the social-behavioral model.

Men like Tony Bennett are extraordinary, but, when you break down the specific elements of their stories, the tactics become clear and the strategies adaptable for all men. Engaging support from loved ones, giving attention to diet and exercise, continuing to work part-time at a job you love, pursuing a passion for learning new skills, improving on your hobbies, and fueling your sense of well-being through the integration of all these factors is a recipe we can all follow. Yes, while Bennett's story is one of inspiration. I'd argue that its greater significance is as an illustration, one of a well-conceived approach to life balanced and anchored in the social-behavioral motivations available to all men.

## Reconnecting

Earlier that same December, I invited the men, I had previously interviewed individually to join me for a group session. I brought 13 of them together to see how they were doing, pose some additional questions, and get their reactions to some specific concepts. As a concluding exercise to my research, I was interested in observing their interactions with each other. I also wanted to see what new insights the group environment might produce.

What I found during the 90-minute session confirmed many of my findings and produced additional stories that support the strength of a social-motivation model in promoting healthy behaviors.

For starters, I witnessed a level of camaraderie among the men. Their common traits, interests, and approaches to life produced a commonality that was evident in their interactions. The men also exhibited what I found to be a high degree of comfort with each other, witnessed by their willingness to share some very personal facts about their health, behavior, and motivation. The interactions were reminiscent of the findings from the Football Fans in Training (FFIT) program and the sense of fraternity among the men reported in that study.

Finally, it was also notable that all 13 of the men, some I hadn't seen in more than a year, still met the criteria for leading a healthy lifestyle consistent with the longevity of healthy behavior found in my survey. While in a non-scientific setting, my observation of this group interaction offers a voice for exploration of the common gender and age as a means to promote initiatives in 50+ men's health.

Going deeper into the dialogue that evening, the feedback offered by the men provided real-life corroborations of how these men keep their values top of mind and carry out a social-behavioral approach to their lives. Here are four stories that aligned directly with my findings and the strategies I've offered:

1. Grandchildren as a motivator.

2. Coping with adversity and the importance of re-engaging in a healthy regimen after living through stressful experiences.

3. Using the social-behavioral model to carry out healthy behaviors.

4. Proactively adjusting to life's hurdles in order to maintain one's exercise routine.

## — Tom —

Tom spoke about a recent exchange with his grandson, who would soon travel to China for a research project. With great pride, he explained how he had taken many trips to China for business during his lifetime, and that his grandson's excursion provided an opportunity for the two of them to spend considerable time together, where Tom could share his experiences. Tom seized the moment to generate some high-quality time with his grandson, which proved to be extremely rewarding for him and a reminder of just how much delight this relationship brings him, "I spent a lot of time with him, showing him where to go and giving him contacts over there. It was something that I owned and was able to give to him. I very much liked that."

## — Alan —

Alan described his experience with a recent diagnosis of kidney cancer. His healthy practices led to early detection and his physical conditioning provided a physical edge in his fight against the disease. He spoke with candor and demonstrated a sense of ease in telling his story to the receptive and supportive group. A real sense of pride came over Alan's face as he described how his doctors acknowledged the value of his physical conditioning in fighting the disease and how he's now cancer-free and back to his exercise:

> I had a slight setback in March. I was diagnosed with kidney cancer, a tumor. They went in and got it out. I'm told I'm cancer free. I'm glad to say that I'm back on the same exercise program that I was prior to the surgery, and I've stepped it up a little bit. I'm really feeling good. I was told that because I was able to have a healthy lifestyle, especially exercise that it helped in the recovery area.

## — Kevin —

Kevin, one of the younger men in the group, shared his experience running his first 5K race with his two preteen sons. It was his first foray into road races, but a venture that offered him a new means to enjoy his parenthood and simultaneously contribute to his physical well-being. He told the men his story with delight, despite what he jokingly characterized as an embarrassing outcome:

> Believe it or not, I've been playing sports my whole life but for the first time, in August or September, I tried my first 5K race and it was brutal. I got though it but my sons crushed me (he said, lovingly), but I'll try another 5K shortly.

## — Robert —

Finally, Robert told us how he brought his dumbbells with him on a business trip to North Carolina, so that he could avoid any inter-ruption to his exercise routine while he was away. He explained that the thought of missing any of his workouts and the challenges of reestablishing his routine were just more than he wanted, and that he was just too wedded to his habits to let something like a business trip to take him off course. Talk about planning ahead and sticking with healthy behaviors:

> My normal routine is to do some work out Monday through Friday: weight lifting, aerobic or something to maintain the routine. I took my weights to the conference so I could maintain the same pattern and didn't have to stop doing it because I was elsewhere.

With a clear and consistent voice, the men's comments added dimension, and reinforcement for the principles of socially driven health behaviors and the outcomes that are achievable through this approach. Their willingness to open up when assembled as a cohort of peers with mutual characteristics and interests is interesting and contributes additional understanding to motivation as a pathway to health. This suggests further study of these dimensions.

## FFIT and EuroFIT in the US

I also took the opportunity to get the men's reaction to the two European-based studies I presented in Chapter 15, Football Fans in Training (FFIT) and EuroFIT. After reviewing the programs with them and showing them photos of potbellied, middle-aged men running around in soccer uniforms, my question was simple: would either of these programs work in the US? If adopted by the National Football League (NFL) or one of the other major professional sports leagues, would men be interested? Is the allegiance of male sports fans to their local teams strong enough to leverage as a bridge to sustainable behavior change?

While there were caveats about costs and other logistics, which I suggested they push aside for the moment, the answer was yes. Their feeling was that American sports fandom has sufficient power to attract the attention of those who would otherwise reject health and fitness and serve as an entrée for the more fitness-challenged among 50+ men. Whether or not governments, such as in Europe, would advance such a concept remained a question among the men, which I consciously deferred to another forum. Nevertheless, I believe that this small sample provided encouragement that such models should receive further consideration for adoption in the US.

Finally, our discussion about engaging the more health-challenged led to an interesting response advanced by Tom and endorsed by some others. To me, it not only serves as a commentary on the task of motivating individual behavior change, but also on my call for broader cultural change.

## Listen for the Opening

Capping the session was a point made by Tom and echoed by Harris and Bob during a conversation about motivating men to live healthily. The discussion highlighted the burden healthy behavior presents for so many men, particularly those over 50. When pressed for their advice, a nuanced, but quite poignant, response came forth.

Tom was quick to acknowledge the difficulty in motivating men to live healthily, a point echoed by the group. However, there was no apprehension toward offering advice for those struggling to adopt better behavior. What did emerge was a strong consensus, identifying receptivity as the biggest hurdle in any attempts to convey the group's positive experience to other men. They noted that many men simply are not interested in a message about health. Good intensions aside, the men were clear: their advice will fall on deaf ears without an openness to listen. With that sentiment as backdrop, Tom offered a suggestion; listen for an opening:

> I try to listen for an opening. Somebody will complain: I had a hard time climbing up the stairs, and then I might say, "It's because you're so heavy, did you ever think about cutting back on food or something like that?" Then they'd say, "Did you do that? Is that how you got where you are?" I'd say, "Yeah, this is what I do and why I can climb a flight of stairs and not get winded." I have found that if you try to go in cold turkey with someone who hasn't indicated they want some help your gonna get stonewalled; they're not gonna listen.

Chiming in, Harris added, "You can listen for the cues. They'll tell you. Wait for that opening. It's a very good point."

Bob's comments highlighted this same "tough love" approach espoused by a number of the men and in my survey, "I'd go for the jugular and ask them: Do you want to be a burden to your family?" To me, that's the biggest risk of aging.

I found these men to be direct, but compassionate. They were realistic about resistance to behavior change, but keenly aware of the potential to break through under the right circumstances: defining moments where the byproducts of poor behaviors manifest themselves or unique situations that highlight the consequences of neglect. Seizing upon these, "moments of acceptance" is a strategy that ties back to the survey findings regarding fear as a motivator. The men in the group understand fear as a lever, but, perhaps more importantly, know precisely when to pull that lever to get the desired response, which is no small point!

## Focusing Events: Timing is Everything!

The group session participants provide deeper insights into the social-based approach to behavior change. Their opinions represent qualitative field-experience that complements the survey's quantitative approach. Their response to the challenge of scaling positive behaviors was of particular significance. Their advice focused primarily on the value of timing and leveraging those unique circumstances that offer an opportunity to break through what they see as substantial impediments to the adoption of behavior change. I would label such circumstances as "focusing events", a term I borrow from my field of public policy, where we used the term to describe events that trigger an immediate policy response (i.e., frequently tragic or stunning events) to issues previously low on the policy agenda.

In the context of men's health, what the men are saying is that you can improve the potential for men to consider behavioral change if we deliver the overture or approximate to a focusing event. This is when the recipient is most likely to accept the message and consider change more seriously. As we have seen from the example offered by Tom, the focusing events need not be tragic, as I have referenced in my policy example (although they can be), but simply enough to connect with a man's fears, the potential for more serious problems should the behavior persist.

I believe that the timing is right for a cultural change in men's health. To have such micro and macro strategies align may be purely coincidental, but I would argue, strategically significant. If timing and the alignment of influencing factors can indeed serve as a tipping point, for individuals or society as a whole, then we need to seize these moments and advance the movement. Whether the focusing event is a man's realization that his pants don't fit or society's recognition that too many men are dying prematurely, the common denominator is a call for action. There is wisdom in the voices of the men who say that you have to "listen for the opening." Their point is pragmatic in terms of individual behavior change, but simultaneously has societal implications well beyond the individual.

## Cultural Change

Geoffrey Canada is an American educator, social activist, and author. Since 1990, Canada has been president of the Harlem Children's Zone, an organization whose goal is to increase high school and college graduation rates among students in Harlem (Gergen, 1998).

Canada is also one of the most motivating speakers I've ever heard. While his message relates to his experience promoting education as a pathway out of poverty and despair for children in Harlem, its application extends much further. The day I was fortunate enough to hear him speak, one of his points hit home with regard to the need for cultural reform for men's health: "Hope is infectious" (Canada, 2016).

Canada's model of grassroots organizing that provides attention to each child, while also promoting systematic reform, is identical to the task facing men's health. Men need a motivational blueprint that enables them to design their individual lifestyle architecture. Concurrently, there is a need for cultural reform within America and our major institutions that will support these individual efforts, causing increasing numbers of men to adopt positive behaviors. Combined, these factors will prompt the spread of hope in an infectious manner.

I remain optimistic as I see the continued spread of hope across our major institutions, each installment inching us closer to the point where healthy behaviors become the norm. Let me offer one final example from the field of medicine.

A study at the Harvard School of Public Health, published in the Journal of the American Medical Association's JAMA Internal Medicine in December, 2016, indicated that female doctors out-performed male doctors, citing that female physicians had lower 30-day mortality than did patients treated by male physicians (Fox, 2016). Beyond the direct importance of the study, its release promoted renewed focus on previous studies that female physicians have a more patient-centered communication style, are more encouraging, and reassuring, and their office visits are longer than male physician's visits are, according to published reports about the study.

What does all this mean? It represents one more installment in a growing consensus of the importance of social determinants in health and the integration of social considerations in shaping health out-comes. It supports the points I have made throughout this book and contributes to the evidence on patient-centered care: the positive outcomes associated with strong social connections between physicians and patients and increased patient engagement.

## You Are in Control

The basis of this book is that behavior has the greatest impact on your health. From that platform, I focused on the sources of motivation for 50+ men, arguing that no diet or exercise program is sustainable without a sufficient and ongoing supply of motivation. My search prompted me to seek out the opinions of those who I deemed the most qualified experts in the field, the 50+ men who lead a healthy lifestyle. Once identified, I embarked on a two-tiered methodology to learn from their experiences, a nationwide survey of 1,000 men and a total of over 30 interviews. The results of these efforts are the underpinnings of a 10-step strategy with exercises, a blueprint for lifestyle architecture.

In the course of braiding the survey data within the stories of the men, I've anchored the dominant themes by providing references from the field of psychology that tie the strategies to well-established, as well as newer, theories to add strength and validity. Complementing the 10 strategies is a discussion of the importance the roles that women and what I call a man's loving constituency play. I conclude with a call for a larger cultural change that is long overdue in this country, citing a unique alignment among three major American institutions, with the advancement of men's health as the basis for this call to action.

While I have employed the stories of two professional athletes and one entertainer, I have most significantly relied on the experiences of everyday men who choose to live healthily in very common ways. Additionally, I shared my personal experiences with health and fitness, and the important role it played in helping me through some tough times as a young, single dad. Simply put, my goal is to convey that if the men in my study and I can successfully employ these strategies, so can you.

Yes, there's reason for hope. Hope that, as an individual or a loving constituent, you can now see a new motivational pathway to health. Hope that the time has come when a healthy lifestyle will become the norm, not the exception, in this nation. Hope that the influential institutions in America will support men's health at much greater levels and, finally, hope that your new healthy lifestyle will bring you all the happiness and fulfillment that awaits.

So, there it is. Now it's up to you. You have the tools. You're in control. I wish you all the best!

# Acknowledgments

BOOK WRITING IS A team sport. In my case, I recruited talented individuals with the technical skills in research, psychology, and storytelling to help me collect data, interpret the results, place them into context, and then translate the findings into easily digestible advice. Anchoring the project team were the healthily behaving men who shared their stories. In doing so, they provided a realistic and emotional element that offers hope to those who aspire to live healthily and enjoy the social benefits of healthy behavior. I feel blessed to have the support of a comprehensive team.

First and foremost is my editor, Cynde Van Patten Christie. Her counsel and guidance kept me focused and diligent in the management of the book when the constraints of a very full-time job and the normal pressures in life required my attention. I offer sincere thanks to Dr. Rachel Pruchno, Rowan University School of Osteopathic Medicine, NJ Institute for Successful Aging, for the introduction to Cynde.

David B. Nash, MD, MBA, Dean of the Thomas Jefferson University School of Population Health provided some early guidance that was invaluable. Also providing counsel on my initial interest in writing a book were my colleagues at Cooper University Health Care, Anthony Mazzarelli, MD, co-president, John Robertson, MD, and Andres Pumariega, MD.

When I decided to pursue the manuscript, a number of individuals played key roles in the development of the research instruments. This included Jill Lawlor at Cooper, Dale Kramer of Kramer Research, John Graham and Randy Hill at Marc Research, and Bethany Farms and Kristen Cuzzo at Plaza Research.

As I embarked on the project Bonnie Joffe at *50 and beyond.com* magazine provided me with a forum to publish several articles based on the initial research results and hone my writing skills. Bob Dalessandro, one of my interviewees, was instrumental in making the connection with Bonnie. My personal physician, Daniel Hyman, DO, division head, Internal Medicine, Department of Medicine, Cooper University Health Care was helpful in offering technical advice for one of these articles.

Another early milestone was my expedition to the University of Rochester, and a meeting with Dr. Edward L. Deci, a major contributor to Self-Determination Theory (SDT). Dr. Deci was gracious in his willingness in allowing me to me interview him and for opening my eyes to the world of SDT and its focus on intrinsic motivation. Through Dr. Deci, I subsequently had the opportunity to meet his colleague Dr. Richard Ryan at the 2016 SDT conference in Victoria Canada, which ultimately led to my connection with Dr. Geoff Williams, a colleague of Deci and Ryan and a practicing physician at the University of Rochester Health Center, Healthy Living Center. Experiencing a patient visit with Dr. Williams, coupled with the ability to interview him, gave me a firsthand look that advanced my understanding of men's health, a huge contribution to this book. The entire team at Rochester was fantastic.

Colleagues at Independence Blue Cross in Philadelphia offered an important perspective on motivation from the view of a major health insurer. My appreciation goes out to Richard Snyder, MD, and his team, Somseh Nigam, and Aaron Smith-McLallen.

Dr. Christopher Nave from the Psychology Department at Rutgers University-Camden was instrumental in providing his academic advice and introducing me to Dr. Kristin August. Dr. August is a health psychologist at Rutgers University-Camden who was incredibly helpful as a sounding board and technical specialist with providing a critique of the manuscript, and in guiding me through the reconciliation of my research and the established principles in health psychology.

She also provided me with opportunities to speak to her students, which I very much enjoyed.

A colleague at the Camden Coalition of Healthcare Providers and MacArthur Fellowship award winner, Dr. Jeffrey Brenner, was another key contributor to this work. I have had the opportunity to work with Dr. Brenner at both Cooper and the Camden Coalition over the years. His thoughts on health and motivation in men were extremely insightful.

While my research included a wide review of the literature and organizations that have contributed to the advancement of men's health, of particular note was the Men's Health Network. Their pioneering work represents important leadership in the field, which was incredibly helpful in building my understanding, particularly in terms of policy-related efforts to improve the state of men's health in our nation.

I could not have completed the book without the hard work of a number of student researchers. They included John Kunkle, Michael Feeney, Ronnie Schmeltzer, Kiersten Westley, and Elisabeth Anne Plotner.

My thanks also extend to the beta readers of this manuscript, who were kind enough to share their feedback and candid observations, which added to the final product. These include Alan Kramer, Dale Kramer, Robert Dalessandro, James Kehoe, Elizabeth Nardi, Dr. Kathleen H. Macfarlane, Rowan University, Ken Shuttleworth, Dr. Christopher Nave, and Dr. Robert Christie.

Kudos as well to all of the men who participated in my national survey, the participants in the focus groups and, in particular, the men who shared their stories in personal interviews, without whom this project would be impossible. Thanks to: Tim S., Bob D., Gautam V., John R., Vijay G., Carmen F., Kevin K., Jay D., David C., Harris S., Thomas D., William B., Rodney C., Robert L., and Alan K. Their stories covey the emotion that lies at the heart of their motivation.

Others at Cooper University Health Care deserve recognition and thanks. My boss, Kevin O'Dowd, co-president and our general counsel, Gary Lesneski, for navigating the requirements of the institution, and our chairman, George Norcross, who has been there for me over my entire career. My appreciation to you all.

Finally, I offer my gratitude to my family and friends who have traveled this journey with me. My wife, Maria, has been a source of support, advice, and inspiration for which I am immensely grateful. My sons, Anthony and Stephen, were more than accommodating in their review of some of my more personally sensitive material. Anthony's support extended to include his professional help in the filming of my interviews with the men. His wife, my daughter-in-law, Colleen, provided her legal expertise, and their son and my grandson, Luca, served a beacon of motivation. My other daughter-in-law, Nicole, was a steady supporter. And, most importantly, my late father, who provided a lifetime of inspiration. He was my hero.

# References

Advisory Board-The Daily Briefing, October 6, 2016.

August, K.J., & Sorkin, D.H. (2011). Support and influence in the context of diabetes management: Do racial/ethnic differences exist? *Journal of Health Psychology*, 16, 711-721. doi: 10.1177/1359105310388320.

Baltes, P.B. (1997). On the incomplete architecture of human ontogeny: Selection, optimization, and compensation as foundation of developmental theory. *American Psychologist 52*(4): 366–380.

Bartholomew, K., & Horowitz, L. M. (1991). Attachment styles among young adults: a test of a four-category model. *Journal of personality and social psychology*, 61(2), 226.

Bates, T. C. (2015). The glass is half-full and half empty: A population-representative twin study testing if optimism and pessimism are distinct systems. *The Journal of Positive Psychology.* doi:10.1080/17439760.2015.1015155.

Beck, A. (1997). The past and the future of cognitive therapy. *Journal of Psychotherapy Practice and Research*, 6, 276-284.

Brandtstädter, J., & Greve, W. (1994). The aging self: Stabilizing and protective processes. *Developmental review, 14*(1), 52-80.

Brandtstädter, J., & Rothermund, K. (1994). Self-percepts of control in middle and later adulthood: buffering losses by rescaling goals. *Psychology and aging, 9*(2), 265.

Brandtstädter, J., Rothermund, K., & Schmitz, U. (1997). Coping resources in later life. *European Review of Applied Psychology/Revue Européenne de Psychologie Appliquée.*

Branstrom, R., Duncan, L.G., Moskowitz, J.T. (2011). The association between dispositional mindfulness, psychological well-being, and perceived health in a Swedish population-based sample.

*British Journal of Health Psychology.* 16 (2): 300–16. doi:10.1348/135910710X501683.

Brott, A., Dougherty, A., Williams, S.T., Matope, J. H., Fadich, A. & Taddelle, M. (2011). The Economic Burden Shouldered by Public and Private Entities as a Consequence of Health Disparities Between Man and Women. *American Journal of Men's Health*, Vol. 5-6, pp.528-539.

Canada, Geoffrey, Speech to the Complex Care Conference, December 9, 2016.

Carrol-Scott, A., Henson, R.M., Kolker, J., Purtle, J. (2017). The Role of Non-Profit Hospitals in Promoting Health Equity in Cities: A Content Analysis of Community Health Needs Assessments and Implementation Strategies. *Journal of Health Affairs.*

Carstensen, L., Isaacowitz, D. & Charles, S. (1999). Taking time seriously: a theory of socioemotional selectivity. *American Psychologist*, 54, 165–81.

Carstensen, Laura. L.
Annual Review of Gerontology and Geriatrics, Volume 11, 1991 Chapter 8 Selectivity Theory: Social Activity in Life-Span Context 1992 Springer Publishing Company, Inc. 536 Broadway, New York, NY 10012-3955

Carver, C. S., Sheier, M. F., & Segerstrom, S. C. (2010). All about Optimism. *Clinical Psychology Review, 30*(7), 879-889. doi:https://doi.org/10.1016/j.cpr.2010.01.006.

Centers for Disease Control and Prevention CDC. (2003). Trends in aging—United States and worldwide. MMWR. *Morbidity and mortality weekly report, 52*(6), 101.

Centers for Disease Control and Prevention. (2015). Basics About Diabetes. Retrieved from https://www.cdc.gov/diabetes/basics/diabetes.html.

Cherry, K. (2016). *The Psychology of Heroism: Are Heroes Born or Made?* Updated July 12, 2016. Retrieved from VeryWell website https://verywell.com/the-psychology-of-heroism-2795905.

Choi, H., Marks, N.F. (2011). Socioeconomic status, marital status continuity and change, marital conflict, and mortality. *Journal of Aging and Health*, 23 (4), pp. 714-742. doi: 10.1177/0898264310393339.

Cohen, S. (2004). Social Relationships and Health. *American Psychologist*.

Corrigan, Janet M., PhD. (2014) Distinguished Fellow, The Dartmouth Institute. Keynote Presentation to the 5th National Accountable Care Organization Summit, June 18, 2014. "Accountable Health Communities Taking Shape" (Power Point Presentation).

Deci, E.L., & Ryan, R.M. (1985b). *Intrinsic Motivation and self-determination in human behavior*. Plenum, New York.

Dionigi, R. A. (2015). Stereotypes of aging: their effects on the health of older adults. *Journal of Geriatrics*, 1(5), 21-22.Dong, X., Milholland, B., & Vijg, J. (2016). Evidence for a limit to human lifespan. *Nature, 538*(7624), 257-259.

Duckworth, A. (2016). *Grit: The power of passion and perseverance*. Simon and Schuster, New York.

Fagundes, C. (2012). Sex, Relationships, and Weight Loss. http://www.webmd.com/diet/obesity/features/sex-relationships-weight-loss#1 Fetters, A. (2014). How to Achieve Runner's High. *Runner's World*.

Fool, M. H. (2014). 50 reasons why this is the greatest time ever. Retrieved March 10, 2017, from http://www.usatoday.com/story/money/personalfinance/2014/02/02/greatest-period-in-history/5161935/.

Fox, M. (2016) NBC News.com *Female Doctors Outperform Male Doctors, According to Study* (2016). December 19. Downloaded 01-02-17.

Galdas, P. M., Cheater, F., & Marshall, P. (2005). Men and health help-seeking behaviour: literature review. *Journal of advanced nursing*, 49(6), 616-623.

Gergen, David (January 20, 1998). "Moving Toward Manhood." PBS. Retrieved 2007-04-24. (Downloaded 1-22-17 Wikipedia)

Giltay, E. J., Geleijnse, J. M., Zitman, F. G., Buijsse, B., & Kromhout, D. (2007). Lifestyle and dietary correlates of dispositional optimism in men: The Zutphen Elderly Study. *Journal of psychosomatic research*, *63*(5), 483-490.

Gremillion, D. (2001). Men's Health Needs a Heartfelt Change. *The News & Observer*, A31.

Health, United States, (2016). Centers for Disease Control and Prevention, National Center for Health Statistics May 2017. DHHS Publication No. 2017-1232

Health, United States, (2016). With Chart book on Long-term Trends in Health. Hyattsville, MD. 2017 Table 57, page 231.

Health, United States, 2016: With Chart book on Long-term Trends in Health. Hyattsville, MD. 2017. Table 45, Page 203.

Hewitt, Aon (2015). *A Business Case for Workers Age 50+ A Look at the Value of Experience 2015*. Retrieved from AARP Website: http://www.aarp.org/research/topics/economics/info-2015/ business-case-older-workers.html.

https://www.goodreads.com/work/quotes/10446115-rocky-balboa. Rocky Balboa Quotes by Silvester Stallone. Downloaded. 8-28-17.

https://www.rpi.edu/dept/advising/american_culture/social_skills/ nonverbal_communication/reading_exercise.htm.

Hunt, K, Wyke, S., Gray, C. M., Anderson, A. S., Brady, A., Bunn, C., Donnan, P.T., Fenwick, E., Grieve, E., Leishman, J., Miller, E., Mutrie, N., Rauchlaus, P., White, A., Treweek, S. (2014). A gender-sensitized weight loss and healthy living programme for overweight and obese men delivered by Scottish Premier League football clubs (FFIT): a pragmatic randomized controlled trial. The Lancet.com, Vol 383, April, 2014. P. 1216, 1218.

Hunt, K., McCann, C., Gray, Mutrie, N. & Wyke, S., (2013). You've got to walk before you run: positive evaluations of a walking program as part of a gender-sensitized, weight-management program delivered to men through professional football clubs. *Health Psychology.* Vol 383, April, 2014. P. 1216, 1218.

Hurd, N. M., Zimmerman, M. A., & Xue, Y. (2009). Negative adult influences and the protective effects of role models: A study with urban adolescents. *Journal of Youth and Adolescence, 38*(6), 777–789. http://doi.org/10.1007/s10964-008-9296-5.

Institute of Medicine (2001). Committee on Health and Behavior: Research, Practice, and Policy. Health and Behavior: The Interplay of Biological, Behavioral, and Societal Influences. *Individuals and Families: Models and Interventions.* https://www.ncbi.nlm.nih.gov/books/NBK43749/\.

Jarrett, C. (2008). *Path of the Golden Heart: Conscious Dating in an Unconscious World* (First Edition ed., Vol. 1). New York, NY: First Edition Design.

Kelloniemi, H., Ek, E., & Laitinen, J. (2005). Optimism, dietary habits, body mass index and smoking among young Finnish adults. *Appetite, 45*(2), 169-176.

Khan, C. M., Stephens, M. A. P., Franks, M. M., Rook, K. S., & Salem, J. K. (2013). Influences of spousal support and control on diabetes management through physical activity. *Health Psychology, 32*, 739–747. doi:10.1037/a0028609.

Kochanek, K., Murphy, S. L., Xu, J., & Tejada-Vera, B. (2016). Deaths: Final Data for 2014. *National Vital Statistics Reports, 65*(4).

Lickerman, A. (2012) *THE UNDEFEATED MIND: On the Science of Constructing an Indestructible Self* (HCI), MD Health Communications, Inc. Deerfield Beach, Florida.

Loprinzi, P. D., et al. (2016). Healthy Lifestyle Characteristics and Their Joint Association With Cardiovascular Disease Biomarkers in US Adults, *Mayo Clinic Proceedings,* Volume 91, Issue 4, 432 – 442. *Atlantic Monthly,* March 23, 2016. Downloaded 9-4-17.

Marchese, J. (2016). "I Just Love What I'm Doing," *New York Times,* December 18, Arts & Leisure Section.

Martins, R. K., & McNeil, D. W. (2009). Review of motivational interviewing in promoting health behaviors. *Clinical Psychology Review*, 29 (4), 283–293. As found in National Registry of evidenced-based Programs and Practices, Literature Review on Motivational Interviewing, downloaded on 9-4-17 from nrepp.samhsa.gov.

Matthews CE, Chen KY, Freedson PS, Buchowski MS, Beech BM, Pate RR, Troiano RP. (2008). Amount of time spent in sedentary behaviors in the United States, 2003–2004. *American Journal of Epidemiology*, 167 (7), 875-881.

McGrath, T. (2007). Why Can't I Get Motivated, *Men's Health*.

Men's Health Network. (2016). Media-NFL Events. www.youtube.com/user/MHNMedia.

Merchant, Nilofer (2011). "Culture Trumps Strategy Every Time." *Harvard Business Review*, March 22, 2011.

Movember Foundation. (2016) About Us. www.us.movember.com/AboutUs.

Murphy. J. (2017). A Fitness Secret: Qigong. *The Wall Street Journal*, p. A12.

Nark, J. (2016). Nearly 80 and still lifting. *Philadelphia Inquirer*, p. B1.

National Center for Chronic Disease Prevention and Health Promotion (NCCD), (2016). Diabetes, Working to Reverse the US Epidemic. *Division of Diabetes Translation*.

Niemiec, C. P., Ryan, R. M., & Deci, E. L. (2009). The path taken: Consequences of attaining intrinsic and extrinsic aspirations in post-college life. *Journal of research in personality*, 43(3), 291-306.

Okun, M.A., Huff, B.P., August, K.J., & Rook, K.S. (2007). Testing hypotheses distilled from four models of the effects of health-related social control. *Basic and Applied Social Psychology*, 29, 185-193. doi: 10.1080/01973530701332245.

Pensiero, N. (2016). Tony Bennett brings 90 years of music to Rowan, *Courier-Post*, December 6, 2016.

Peters, T., & Waterman, R. H. (1982). In Search of Excellence: Lessons from America's Best Run Companies.

Pink, D. H. (2011). *Drive: The surprising truth about what motivates us.* Penguin, London, England.

Ragin Fish, D. (2015). Health Psychology. Pearson Education, Inc. Second Edition. Pg. 169-175.

Rasmussen, H.N., Scheier, M.F. & Greenhouse, J.B. (2009) Optimism and physical health: A meta-analytic review. Annals of Behavioral Medicine. 37: 239. doi:10.1007/s12160-009-9111-.

Report to the President (2016). *Independence, Technology, and Connection in Older Age Executive Office of the President President's Council of Advisors on Science and Technology,* March 2016, Executive Summary.

Rius-Ottenheim, N., Kromhout, D., Mast, R. C., Zitman, F. G., Geleijnse, J. M., & Giltay, E. J. (2011). Dispositional optimism and loneliness in older men. *International Journal of Geriatric Psychiatry, 27*(2), 151-159. doi:10.1002/gps.2701

Rothermund, K., & Brandtstadter, J. (2003). Coping with deficits and losses in later life: From compensatory action to accommodation. *Psychology and aging, 18*(4), 896-905.

Rothman, A. J., & Salovey, P. (1997). Shaping perceptions to motivate healthy behavior: The role of message framing. *Psychological Bulletin,* 121(1), 3-19. doi:10.1037//0033-2909.121.1.3

Ryan, R. M., Deci, E.L., (2011). Self-Determination Theory and the Facilitation of Intrinsic Motivation, Social Development, and Well-Being. *American Psychologist,* 55(1), 68.

Sabir, M. (2015). Personalized and global generativity: A prevalent, important, but unlabeled distinction in the literature. *Journal of Adult Development,* 22(1), 14-26.

Sandman, D., Simantov, E. & and An, C., (2000). The Commonwealth Fund, March 2000. *Out of Touch: American Men and the Health Care System.*

Saxbe, D. E. (2008). Marital satisfaction, recovery from work, and diurnal cortisol among men and women. *Health Psychology*, Vol 27(1), Jan 2008, 15-25.

Schroder, S. A. (2007). We Can Do Better—Improving the Health of the American People. *New England Journal of Medicine*.

Schulman, P.; Keith, D.; Seligman, M. (1993). "Is Optimism Heritable? A Study of Twins". *Behavior Research and Therapy* 31 (6): 569–574. doi:10.1016/0005-7967(93)90108-7.

Seligman, M. E. P. (2006). *Learned optimism: How to change your mind and your life.* New York: Vintage Books.

Silva, M. (2016). The Power of football: Using self-determination theory to promote health behavior change in the European Fans in Training (EuroFIT) project. Presentation at the Self-Determination Theory Conference, June, 2016.

Smith-McLallen, A. (2013). https://www.linkedin.com/in/aaron-smith-mclallen-7418b62b, accessed October 30, 2016.

Smith-McLallen, A. (2015). Changing Health Behavior. *Theory and Practice*.

Squires, D. & Anderson, C. (2015). *U.S. Health Care from a Global Perspective: Spending, Use of Services, Prices, and Health in 13 Countries.* The Commonwealth Fund.

Steptoe, A., Wright, C., Kunz-Ebrecht, S. R., & Iliffe, S. (2006). Dispositional optimism and health behaviour in community-dwelling older people: Associations with healthy ageing. *British journal of health psychology, 11*(1), 71-84.

The Advisory Board, (2016). Aging Well in the 21st Century: Strategic Directions for Research on Aging, *National Institute on Aging*.

The Pew Research Center, (2014). Number of older Americans in the workforce is on the rise.

The State of Obesity 2017, Trust for America's Health, Washington, D.C., August 31, 2017. https://www.tfah.org/releases/stateofobesity2017/

Trust for America's Health is a non-profit, non-partisan organization dedicated to saving lives by protecting the health of every community and working to make disease prevention a national priority. For more information, visit www.healthyamericans.org.

For more than 40 years the Robert Wood Johnson Foundation has worked to improve health and health care. We are striving to build a national Culture of Health that will enable all to live longer, healthier lives now and for generations to come. For more information, visit www.rwjf.org. Follow the Foundation on Twitter at www.rwjf.org/twitter or on Facebook at www.rwjf.org/facebook.

Toossi, M. (2013) "Labor force projections to 2022: the labor force participation rate continues to fall," *Monthly Labor Review,* U.S. Bureau of Labor Statistics, https://doi.org/10.21916/mlr.2013.40.

Trief, P. M., Sandberg, J., Greenberg, R. P., Graff, K., Castronova, N., Yoon, M, Weinstock, R. S. (2003). Describing support: A qualitative study of couples living with diabetes. *Families, Systems, & Health,* 21, 57–67. doi:10.1037/h0089502.

Troiano, B., Berrigan, D., Dodd, K., Mâsse, C. Tilert, T. & McDowell, M. (2008). Physical activity in the United States measured by accelerometer. *U.S. National Library of Medicine Medical Science Sports Exercise.* 40(1):181-8.

Tucker, J. S., & Anders, S. L. (2001). Social control of health behaviors in marriage. *Journal of Applied Social Psychology,* 31, 467–485. doi: 10.1111/j.1559-1816.2001.tb02051.x.

Twenge, Jean M., (2015). Are Mental Health Issues on the Rise? *Psychology Today.* Posted 10-12-15. Downloaded 9-4-17.

US Department of Health and Human Services. (1990). Healthy People 2000: National Health Promotion and Disease Prevention Objectives-Nutrition Priority Area. *Nutrition Today,* 25(6), 29-39.

Wakefield, J. C. (1998). Immortality and the externalization of the self: Plato's unrecognized theory of generativity. *American Psychological Association.* (pp. 133–174).

Waldinger, R. (2015, November). Robert Waldinger: What makes a good life? Lessons from the longest study on happiness [Video file]. Retrieved from https://www.ted.com/talks/waldinger_robert_ What makes a good life? Lessons from the longest study on happiness.

Walsh, J. (2016). Campbell Soup backs venture in Nutrition. *Courier-Post.*

Web site About FFIT, ffit.org.UK/page 11, Referenced 10-15-2016.

Webb, T.L., & Sheehan, P. (2006) Does changing behavioral intentions engender behavior change? A meta-analysis of the experimental evidence. Centers for Medicare & Medicaid Services, CMS.Gov 2016 *Psychological Bulletin* (132(2) 249-.

Werner, E. E. (1995). Resilience in development. *Current directions in psychological science, 4*(3), 81-84 What is Cognitive Behavior Therapy (CBT) https://www.beckinstitute.org/about-beck/our-history/, Accessed February 19, 2017.

Werner, E. E. (1995). Resilience in Development. *Current directions in psychological science, 4*(3), 81–84. https://doi.org/10.1111/1467-8721.ep10772327

White, Gazewood, & Mounsey, 2007). *Medical Teacher* Vol. 29, Issue. 4, 2007, Pages e67-e71 | Published online: 03 Jul 2009.

Xu, K. T., & Borders, T. F. (2003). Gender, health, and physician visits among adults in the United States. *American journal of public health,* 93(7), 1076-1079.

Yancey, A. K., Siegel, J. M., & McDaniel, K. L. (2002). Role models, ethnic identity, and health-risk behaviors in urban adolescents. *Archives of Pediatrics & Adolescent Medicine, 156*(1), 55-61.

# About the Author

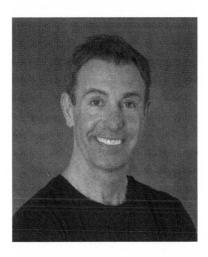

Louis Bezich is a healthcare executive, husband, father, grandfather, part-time professor, and author with a passion for health and fitness. His devotion is a result of a lifetime of experiences that included divorce, single parenthood, and professional challenges where diet and exercise became the antidote that carried him though the tough times and ultimately enabled him to flourish personally and professionally. Decades later, what started as a coping mechanism for an ambitious twenty-something has grown into a commitment that drives this sixty-something to share his experience, promote social motivation models, and advocate for a new culture of men's health.

An executive for over 40 years in the public and private sectors, Bezich currently serves as a Senior Vice-President with Cooper University Health Care and is an adjunct professor in the Graduate Department of Public Policy and Administration at the Camden Campus of Rutgers University. He also sits on various public, non-profit and corporate boards.

Bezich has published numerous articles in the field of public administration and health. He is also contributing author to *Corporate*

*Lawbreaking and Interactive Compliance,* edited by Jay A. Sigler and Joseph E. Murphy. He holds a master's degree in public policy from Rutgers University, a bachelor's degree in social science from the University of Tampa and is a graduate of Harvard University's Program for Senior Executives in State and Local Government.

*CRACK THE CODE: 10 Proven Secrets that Motivate Healthy Behavior and Inspire Fulfillment in Men Over 50* is his first book.

# Index

Made in the USA
Middletown, DE
07 August 2019